# Immunotherapy in Cancer

*Editor*

PATRICK A. OTT

# HEMATOLOGY/ONCOLOGY CLINICS OF NORTH AMERICA

www.hemonc.theclinics.com

*Consulting Editors*
GEORGE P. CANELLOS
H. FRANKLIN BUNN

April 2019 • Volume 33 • Number 2

**ELSEVIER**

1600 John F. Kennedy Boulevard • Suite 1800 • Philadelphia, Pennsylvania, 19103-2899

http://www.theclinics.com

**HEMATOLOGY/ONCOLOGY CLINICS OF NORTH AMERICA Volume 33, Number 2**
**April 2019 ISSN 0889-8588, ISBN 13: 978-0-323-67904-6**

Editor: Stacy Eastman
Developmental Editor: Kristen Helm

*Hematology/Oncology Clinics* (ISSN 0889-8588) is published bimonthly by Elsevier Inc., 360 Park Avenue South, New York, NY 10010-1710. Months of issue are February, April, June, August, October, and December. Business and Editorial Offices: 1600 John F. Kennedy Blvd., Ste. 1800, Philadelphia, PA 19103—2899. Customer Service Office: 3251 Riverport Lane, Maryland Heights, MO 63043. Periodicals postage paid at New York, NY and at additional mailing offices. Subscription prices are $430.00 per year (domestic individuals), $830.00 per year (domestic institutions), $100.00 per year (domestic students/residents), $480.00 per year (Canadian individuals), $1028.00 per year (Canadian institutions) $547.00 per year (international individuals), $1028.00 per year (international institutions), and $255.00 per year (international and Canadian students/residents). International air speed delivery is included in all *Clinics* subscription prices. All prices are subject to change without notice. **POSTMASTER:** Send address changes to *Hematology/Oncology Clinics of North America*, Elsevier Health Sciences Division, Subscription Customer Service, 3251 Riverport Lane, Maryland Heights, MO 63043. Customer Service (orders, claims, online, change of address): Elsevier Health Sciences Division, Subscription **Customer Service, 3251 Riverport Lane, Maryland Heights, MO 63043. Tel: 1-800-654-2452 (U.S. and Canada); 314-447-8871 (outside U.S. and Canada). Fax: 314-447-8029. E-mail: journalscustomerservice-usa@elsevier.com (for print support)**; **journalsonlinesupport-usa@elsevier.com (for online support)**.

*Reprints.* For copies of 100 or more, of articles in this publication, please contact the Commercial Reprints Department, Elsevier Inc., 360 Park Avenue South, New York, New York 10010-1710; Tel.: 212-633-3874, Fax: 212-633-3820, E-mail: reprints@elsevier.com.

*Hematology/Oncology Clinics of North America* is covered in *MEDLINE/PubMed (Index Medicus), EMBASE/ Excerpta Medica, and BIOSIS.*

# Contributors

## CONSULTING EDITORS

**GEORGE P. CANELLOS, MD**
William Rosenberg Professor of Medicine, Department of Medical Oncology, Dana-Farber Cancer Institute, Boston, Massachusetts, USA

**H. FRANKLIN BUNN, MD**
Professor of Medicine, Division of Hematology, Brigham and Women's Hospital, Harvard Medical School, Boston, Massachusetts, USA

## EDITOR

**PATRICK A. OTT, MD, PhD**
Associate Professor of Medicine, Harvard Medical School, Clinical Director, Melanoma Center & Center for Immuno-Oncology, Dana-Farber Cancer Institute, Department of Medicine, Brigham and Women's Hospital, Boston, Massachusetts, USA; Broad Institute of MIT and Harvard, Cambridge, Massachusetts, USA

## AUTHORS

**LUKE W. BARKER, BS**
Medical Student, College of Physicians and Surgeons, Columbia University Irving Medical Center, New York, New York, USA

**RICHARD BRYAN BELL, MD, DDS, FACS**
Medical Director, Head and Neck Surgical Oncologist, Earle A. Chiles Research Institute, Robert W. Franz Cancer Center, Providence Portland Medical Center, Providence Cancer Institute, Head and Neck Institute, Portland, Oregon, USA

**MARIJO BILUSIC, MD, PhD**
Genitourinary Malignancies Branch, Center for Cancer Research, National Cancer Institute, National Institutes of Health, Bethesda, Maryland, USA

**DARIUS D. BORDBAR, BS**
Medical Student, College of Physicians and Surgeons, Columbia University Irving Medical Center, New York, New York, USA

**ELIZABETH I. BUCHBINDER, MD**
Instructor in Medicine, Department of Medical Oncology, Dana-Farber Cancer Institute, Harvard Medical School, Boston, Massachusetts, USA

**PETER DÜWELL, PhD**
Institute of Innate Immunity, University of Bonn, Bonn, Germany

**PETER J. DEMARIA, MD**
Genitourinary Malignancies Branch, Center for Cancer Research, National Cancer Institute, National Institutes of Health, Bethesda, Maryland, USA

**CAMDEN L. ESANCY, MS**
Research Technician, Department of Medicine, Columbia University Irving Medical Center, New York, New York, USA

**GRACE G. FINKEL, BA**
Medical Student, College of Physicians and Surgeons, Columbia University Irving Medical Center, New York, New York, USA

**ROBYN D. GARTRELL, MD**
Postdoctoral Research Fellow, Department of Medicine, Columbia University Irving Medical Center, New York, New York, USA

**SIMON HEIDEGGER, MD**
Medizinische Klinik und Poliklinik 3, Klinikum rechts der Isar, Technische Universität München, Munich, Germany

**SEBASTIAN KOBOLD, MD**
Member of the German Center of Lung Research, Division of Clinical Pharmacology, Center of Integrated Protein Science Munich (CIPS-M), Klinikum der Universität München, Munich, Germany

**GEOFFREY Y. KU, MD**
Gastrointestinal Oncology Service, Department of Medicine, Memorial Sloan Kettering Cancer Center, New York, New York, USA

**JONATHAN E. LEEMAN, MD**
Department of Radiation Oncology, Dana-Farber Cancer Institute, Brigham and Women's Hospital, Boston, Massachusetts, USA

**ROM LEIDNER, MD**
Medical Oncologist, Earle A. Chiles Research Institute, Robert W. Franz Cancer Center, Providence Portland Medical Center, Providence Cancer Institute, Portland, Oregon, USA

**CHARLENE M. MANTIA, MD**
Division of Hematology and Oncology, Beth Israel Deaconess Medical Center, Harvard Medical School, Boston, Massachusetts, USA

**KIM MARGOLIN, MD**
Professor, Department of Medical Oncology, City of Hope National Medical Center, Duarte, California, USA

**PATRICK A. OTT, MD, PhD**
Associate Professor of Medicine, Harvard Medical School, Clinical Director, Melanoma Center & Center for Immuno-Oncology, Dana-Farber Cancer Institute, Department of Medicine, Brigham and Women's Hospital, Boston, Massachusetts, USA; Broad Institute of MIT and Harvard, Cambridge, Massachusetts, USA

**EMANUELLE M. RIZK, BA**
Research Technician, Department of Medicine, Columbia University Irving Medical Center, New York, New York, USA

**YVONNE M. SAENGER, MD**
Florence Irving Assistant Professor of Medicine, Department of Medicine, Columbia University Irving Medical Center, New York, New York, USA

**JONATHAN D. SCHOENFELD, MD, MPhil, MPH**
Department of Radiation Oncology, Dana-Farber Cancer Institute, Brigham and Women's Hospital, Boston, Massachusetts, USA

**ANN W. SILK, MD, MS**
Member of Faculty, Rutgers Cancer Institute of New Jersey, New Brunswick, New Jersey, USA; Dana-Farber Cancer Institute, Boston, Massachusetts, USA

**FELIX SIM, MBBS, BDS, FRACDS(OMS)**
Department of Oral and Maxillofacial Surgery, The Royal Melbourne Hospital, Parkville, Victoria, Australia; Department of Oral and Maxillofacial Surgery, Monash Health, Bentleigh East, Victoria, Australia; Oral and Maxillofacial Surgery Unit, Barwon Health, Geelong, Victoria, Australia

# Contents

Cancer vaccines are a promising strategic approach within the rapidly growing field of immuno-oncology. Therapeutic cancer vaccines are distinct from prophylactic vaccines and vary by both target antigen and vaccine platform. There are currently 3 FDA-approved therapeutic cancer vaccines: intravesical BCG live, sipuleucel-T, and T-VEC. Prior clinical trials have shown that vaccines are generally well tolerated, exhibit unique kinetics, can target tumor neoantigens, and induce antigen cascade. Ongoing clinical trials seek to improve vaccine efficacy either by targeting novel antigens or by combining vaccines with standard-of-care therapies or other immune therapies.

The innate immune system has evolved as a first line of defense against invading pathogens and acts via classes of germline-encoded receptor systems to respond with proinflammatory cytokines. Innate immune cells, predominantly cells of the myeloid compartment, are capable of providing a potent basis for boosting adaptive immunity in malignant diseases. The authors review their current understanding of the molecular mechanisms whereby innate pattern recognition receptors participate in immunosurveillance of cancer cells. They discuss how innate effector mechanisms are currently being targeted pharmacologically and how improved understanding of the biology of these pathways is leading to novel immunotherapies of cancer.

Radiotherapy has known immunomodulatory effects and there exists a strong preclinical rationale for combining radiotherapy with immunotherapies. Broadly, the concurrent administration of immunotherapies and radiotherapy does not seem to result in undue toxicity, even when radiotherapy is administered to definitive doses. Recently reported results from prospective clinical trials evaluating radiotherapy/ICB combinations, such as the PACIFIC trial, provide important information on safety and efficacy in the definitive setting and identify potential abscopal effects. This review details the preclinical foundation for the combination of radiotherapy and immunotherapies, summarizes the most recent clinical data available, and highlights active and future areas of study.

Melanoma and other solid cancers with low or absent T-cell inflammation respond poorly to immune checkpoint inhibitors. Tumor infiltration with T cells that are directed against tumor antigens requires the induction of an innate immune response leading to production of type I interferons and maturation and activation of dendritic cells that can cross-present tumor antigens to T cells. Intralesional therapies, including oncolytic viral therapies, inflammatory cytokines, and agonists of Toll-like receptors and stimulator of interferon genes, can provide the necessary stimuli to trigger such an innate immune response.

The processes controlled by cytokines may be co-opted by pathologic states, contributing to processes that threaten host well-being. A nuanced understanding of this immense web of chemical communications will allow us to understand the mechanisms and limitations of current therapies and to enhance their therapeutic benefits while minimizing their toxicities. This article reviews the current state of cytokine science in malignancy, focusing on agents that are approved for therapy or are in late-stage development. Promising new directions, including novel engineered.

The development of immunotherapy to target cancer has led to improved treatment of many types of malignancy. The immune checkpoint inhibitors are a class of medications that block cell signaling and allow the immune system to recognize and attack cancer cells. CTLA-4, PD-1, and PD-L1 inhibitors have been approved as treatment options in many different types of localized and advanced malignancies. Immune checkpoint inhibitors can be associated with unique side effects known as immune-related adverse events. Side effects most commonly occur in the skin, gastrointestinal tract, lung, and endocrine glands but can affect other organ systems as well.

Immunotherapy has drastically improved the prognosis of many patients with cancer, but it can also lead to severe immune-related adverse events. Biomarkers, which are molecular markers that indicate a patient's disease outcome or a patient's response to treatment, are therefore crucial to helping clinicians weigh the potential benefits of immunotherapy against its potential toxicities. Immunohistochemistry (IHC) has thus far been a powerful technique for discovery and use of biomarkers such as CD8$^+$ tumor-infiltrating lymphocytes. However, IHC has limited reproducibility. Thus, if more IHC-based biomarkers are to reach the clinic, refinement of the technique using multiplexing or automation is key.

## Special Articles

The immune system has a vital role in the development, establishment, and progression of head and neck squamous cell carcinoma (HNSCC). Immune evasion of cancer cells leads to progression of HNSCC. An understanding of this mechanism provides the basis for improved therapies and outcomes for patients. Through the tumor's influence on the microenvironment, the immune system can be exploited to promote metastasis, angiogenesis, and growth. This article provides an overview of the interaction between immune infiltrating cells in the tumor microenvironment, and the immunologic principles related to HNSCC. Current immunotherapeutic strategies and emerging results from ongoing clinical trials are presented.

This review summarizes completed and ongoing studies evaluating the activity of immune checkpoint inhibitors in esophagogastric cancer.

# HEMATOLOGY/ONCOLOGY CLINICS OF NORTH AMERICA

---

**SERIES OF RELATED INTEREST**

*Surgical Oncology Clinics of North America*

---

**THE CLINICS ARE AVAILABLE ONLINE!**
Access your subscription at:
www.theclinics.com

# Preface

# Immunotherapy: An Old and New Modality for the Treatment of Cancer

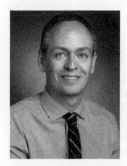

Patrick A. Ott, MD, PhD
*Editor*

Employing a patient's own immune system for the treatment of cancer has been a promise for more than a century. Antibodies targeting programmed death 1 and other inhibitory receptors expressed on T cells, cancer cells, and other immune cells have demonstrated antitumor activity across solid and hematologic malignancies, leading to a number of approvals by regulatory agencies. These antibodies, also called immune checkpoint inhibitors (ICIs), can achieve durable tumor responses, sometimes lasting several years. Because of these recent successes, immunotherapy has taken center stage in the development of new treatments for cancer. While the broad activity of ICI provides proof of principle for the efficacy of cancer immunotherapy, ICIs, at least in monotherapy, have limitations as evident by the relatively low response rates in most cancers, the lack of complete responses in the majority of patients, and the absence of meaningful efficacy in several common malignancies, including prostate, colon, and pancreatic cancer. An effective anticancer immune response comprises multiple components, as illustrated by the Cancer Immunity Cycle. This reality is challenging and likely explains at least in part the heterogeneity of therapeutic success with a given therapy (such as ICIs); however, it also affords many opportunities for therapeutic manipulation since each component of the cancer immune response is a potential target for therapeutic intervention. Many immunotherapeutic strategies, including cancer vaccines, cytokines, and toll-like receptor agonists, had already been tested quite extensively prior to the emergence of ICIs. Given the renewed prominence of immunotherapy stimulated by ICIs, these approaches and many others are now being tested, often in combination with ICIs. The emergence of immunotherapy as a new

Hematol Oncol Clin N Am 33 (2019) xi–xii
https://doi.org/10.1016/j.hoc.2019.01.001
0889-8588/19/© 2019 Published by Elsevier Inc.

modality for cancer therapy comes at a fortuitous time: Recent technological advances have vastly expanded our knowledge of cancer biology, allowing ever more rigorous clinical investigation.

In this issue of *Hematology/Oncology Clinics of North America*, a number of immunotherapeutic strategies are reviewed by leaders in the field. In addition, immune-related toxicities mediated by ICIs and biomarkers for cancer immunotherapy are highlighted by outstanding groups of experts. Drs DeMaria and Bilusic present an in-depth review of the field of cancer vaccines. Dr Düwell, Heidegger, and Kobold review our current knowledge of the molecular mechanisms that trigger innate immune responses and how these insights can be employed to stimulate innate immunity in order to maximize the potential of an adaptive immune response against cancer. In the article, "Radiation Therapy and Immune Modulation," Drs Leeman and Schoenfeld discuss the preclinical rationale and emergent clinical evidence supporting combined radiotherapy and immunotherapy for the treatment of cancer. In the article, "Intralesional Cancer Immunotherapies," I examine the rapidly expanding approach of locally injecting agents that can trigger innate immunity and/or directly kill cancer cells, including oncolytic viruses, Toll-like receptor agonists, and cytokines. Drs Silk and Margolin examine cytokines for the treatment of cancer, including approved drugs, such as interferon-$\alpha$ and interleukin-2, as well as agents in clinical development and novel constructs. Drs Mantia and Buchbinder review the pathophysiology, clinical presentation, and management of immune-related toxicities, and Drs Rizk, Gartrell, Barker, Esancy, Finkel, Bordbar, and Saenger explore prognostic and predictive immunohistochemistry-based biomarkers in cancer and immunotherapy.

I hope that this issue will contribute to the education of students and clinical investigators and help to advance the field of cancer immunotherapy.

Patrick A. Ott, MD, PhD
Melanoma Center & Center for Immuno-Oncology
Dana Farber Cancer Institute
Harvard Medical School
450 Brookline Avenue
Boston, MA 02215-5450, USA

*E-mail address:*
Patrick_Ott@DFCI.harvard.edu

# Cancer Vaccines

Peter J. DeMaria, MD[a],*, Marijo Bilusic, MD, PhD[b]

## KEYWORDS

- Cancer immunotherapy • Immuno-oncology • Vaccine • Cancer vaccine
- Therapeutic cancer vaccine • Antigen cascade

## KEY POINTS

- Therapeutic cancer vaccines are a promising immunotherapeutic treatment modality; however, it is unlikely that cancer vaccines given alone can dramatically change cancer outcomes.
- Multiple clinical trials have shown that vaccines are well tolerated and safe.
- Cancer vaccines can induce antigen cascade or epitope spreading, effecting a distant and durable immune response.
- Ongoing clinical trials seek to improve cancer vaccine efficacy by targeting novel antigens and by combining cancer vaccines with standard-of-care treatments and other immuno-oncology agents with the goal of generating future immune-based platforms.
- Development of successful immune-based platforms will require randomized clinical trials investigating vaccine combinations, treatment sequence, and new biomarkers of immune response.

## INTRODUCTION

Cancer immunotherapy, or immuno-oncology, is a rapidly growing field of cancer research dedicated to developing novel cancer therapies by understanding and harnessing immune pathways. Whereas twentieth-century oncology was transformed by the discovery of cytotoxic chemotherapy and, later, targeted agents, the first systematic study of immuno-oncology predated the discovery of nitrogen mustards and folic acid antagonists by 4 decades.[1]

Disclosure Statement: The authors have no relevant affiliations or financial involvement with any organization or entity with a financial interest in or financial conflict with the subject matter or materials discussed in the article. This includes employment, consultancies, honoraria, stock ownership or options, expert testimony, grants or patents received or pending, or royalties.

[a] Genitourinary Malignancies Branch, Center for Cancer Research, National Cancer Institute, National Institutes of Health, 10 Center Drive, Building 10, Room B2L312, Bethesda, MD 20892, USA; [b] Genitourinary Malignancies Branch, Center for Cancer Research, National Cancer Institute, National Institutes of Health, 10 Center Drive, Building 10, Room B2L324B, Bethesda, MD 20892, USA
* Corresponding author.
E-mail address: peter.demaria@nih.gov

In 1891, Dr William B. Coley, the "Father of Immunotherapy," noted the beneficial effect of erysipelas and fever on malignant tumors.[2] In his capacity as chief bone surgeon at Memorial Hospital in New York, Coley inoculated sarcoma patients with *Streptococcus pyogenes* and *Serratia marcescens*.[3–5] Interest in Coley's primitive cancer vaccine waxed and waned until a 1962 controlled study by Johnston and Novales[6] posthumously validated Coley when his immune-stimulating inoculations generated a 20% response rate. Studies in subsequent decades have further validated Coley's work, and many immune therapies are now approved by the US Food and Drug Administration (FDA). This review provides an overview of the basic principles behind contemporary vaccine development and the future of therapeutic vaccine research.

## HISTORICAL ORIGINS OF VACCINATION

The term "vaccine" is derived from the Latin "vacca," or cow, a reference to the English physician Edward Jenner's original cowpox vaccine. In 1796, Jenner extracted fluid from a cowpox pustule on the hand of an infected milkmaid and inoculated a healthy 8-year-old boy with the fluid. When the boy was variolated with smallpox shortly thereafter, he did not develop the disease.[7] Jenner's case series of 10 successfully vaccinated patients[8] paved the way for the modern era of vaccination, culminating 2 centuries later with the World Health Organization's 1979 declaration of the global eradication of smallpox.[9]

## PROPHYLACTIC VERSUS THERAPEUTIC VACCINES

Cancer vaccines are subclassified as either therapeutic or prophylactic interventions. Prophylactic vaccines are forms of primary and secondary cancer prevention, aimed at reducing cancer incidence, morbidity, and mortality. Prophylactic cancer vaccines have proved successful for the primary prevention of hepatocellular carcinoma secondary to hepatitis B virus and squamous cell carcinoma secondary to human papillomavirus (HPV). Whereas prophylactic vaccines such as Jenner's cowpox vaccine are given to healthy people to prevent future disease,[10] therapeutic vaccines are given to treat existing malignancy. It is noteworthy that adjuvant vaccination strategies intended to prevent relapse or metastatic disease are considered therapeutic, despite their technical designation as tertiary cancer prevention.[10]

## VACCINE TARGETS

Therapeutic cancer vaccines can target a spectrum of antigens expressed by tumor cells. The first cancer vaccines used whole-cell preparations administered in combination with an adjuvant or virus to generate an enhanced immune response. Recent research has uncovered a wide variety of potential targets for cancer vaccines. Newer vaccines target tumor-specific antigens (TSAs), which are uniquely expressed in tumor cells, or tumor-associated antigens (TAAs), which are expressed at low levels in both tumor cells and healthy cells.[11] Well-known targets include mutated oncoproteins such as p53, ras, and B-Raf that result from point mutations and fusions. There are overexpressed antigens such as mucin 1 (MUC1) and human epidermal growth factor receptor (EGFR), and oncofetal antigens such as carcinoembryonic antigen (CEA) and α-fetoprotein. Viral antigens associated with HPV and hepatitis viruses can be targeted, as can tissue lineage and differentiation antigens such as prostatic acid phosphatase (PAP), prostate-specific antigen (PSA), glycoprotein 100 (gp100), and melanoma antigen recognized by T cells 1 (MART-1).[12] Cancer-testis (CT) antigens are promising targets expressed in male germ cells in healthy adults and in multiple cancer types.[13] CT antigens under investigation include melanoma-associated antigen 1 (MAGE-1) and New York esophageal carcinoma antigen 1 (NY-ESO-1). Vascular endothelial growth factor receptor-directed vaccines can target the tumor microenvironment.[14] Vaccines can also target cancer stem cells and interrupt the process of invasion and metastasis via recently discovered antigens such as brachyury, a driver of epithelial-mesenchymal transition.[15] In addition to TSAs and TAAs, personalized therapeutic cancer vaccines, as monotherapy or in combination with other therapies,[16] can immunize patients against their own neoepitopes (mutated antigens produced by an individual tumor). This can eventually activate effector T cells and kill tumors.

## VACCINE PLATFORMS

Current cancer vaccines vary not only by target antigens and immune adjuvants, but also by vaccine platforms, including such broad platforms as peptides/proteins, whole tumor cells, recombinant vectors, dendritic cells (DCs), gangliosides, and genes. Each has advantages and disadvantages.

The most common vaccine platform is peptides/proteins. These vaccines are relatively simple and economical to develop. However, the simplicity of a platform may prove problematic if its short amino acid sequence fails to encode sufficient antigenic material to induce an immune response. Thus, peptide vaccines usually require an immune adjuvant. Given their larger amino acid sequence, protein vaccines are more costly to produce than peptide vaccines, but they may provoke a stronger response.[17] Both peptide and protein vaccines are population-restricted by human leukocyte antigen.

Whole tumor-cell vaccines, subclassified as either autologous or allogeneic,[18] can present a wide variety of TAAs. This lack of specificity may dilute the immune response, however, necessitating additional stimulation via granulocyte-macrophage colony-stimulating factor (GM-CSF) or bacillus Calmette-Guérin (BCG). Autologous vaccines, first tested in 1978,[19] are typically irradiated and require an adjuvant.[20] Autologous vaccines require tumor procurement from the patient, which is not always feasible. GM-CSF-transduced autologous tumor-cell vaccines have been investigated extensively, but none is currently FDA approved.[21] Allogeneic whole tumor-cell vaccines contain several established malignant cell lines, offering an unlimited supply of tumor antigen at reduced cost. However, promising phase II studies have been followed by negative phase III trials, so that no allogeneic whole tumor-cell vaccine is currently FDA approved.[22]

Recombinant poxvirus vaccines are reportedly safe and can express substantial amounts of foreign DNA. Numerous ongoing trials are investigating recombinant vectors, most using modified poxviruses such as vaccinia or avipoxvirus. The immunogenic efficacy of vaccinia is self-limiting, however, and the host generally neutralizes the virus after one or two vaccinations.[12]

DCs are professional antigen-presenting cells (APCs) that activate T lymphocytes through major histocompatibility complex (MHC) signaling.[23] Autologous DC vaccines can be pulsed with peptide or protein or infected with a viral vector. DC vaccines require complicated preparation, but the platform has proved successful. In 2010, the FDA approved sipuleucel-T (PROVENGE®) for metastatic castration-resistant prostate cancer (mCRPC).[24]

Gangliosides are glycolipids that are overexpressed in several tumor types.[25] Although ganglioside-targeting monoclonal antibodies (dinutuximab) are FDA approved,[26] prior phase III clinical trials of vaccine monotherapies targeting these tumor antigens were negative.[27,28]

Genetic vaccines use viral or plasmid vectors to transfect RNA or DNA into host somatic cells that directly produce the desired target antigen. DNA vaccination has proved simple, stable, cost-effective, and safe. The platform is, however, limited by weak immunogenicity through a strong host cellular immune response and will likely require additional priming techniques to be successful.[29]

## APPROVED THERAPEUTIC CANCER VACCINES

Therapeutic cancer vaccines are currently FDA approved for the treatment of early-stage bladder cancer, mCRPC, and metastatic melanoma.

### TheraCys® and TICE®

TheraCys (intravesical BCG live; Sanofi Pasteur) was approved by the FDA in 1990 for intravesical use in the treatment and prophylaxis of urothelial carcinoma in situ of the urinary bladder and for prophylaxis of primary or recurrent stage Ta and/or T1 urothelial carcinoma following transurethral resection.[30] A multicenter, randomized, open-label, phase III trial comparing intravesical BCG vaccine and intravesical doxorubicin demonstrated a 5-year disease-free survival of 45% for BCG recipients versus 18% for doxorubicin recipients.[31] The therapeutic benefit of BCG vaccine was confirmed by a subsequent meta-analysis that showed a 27% reduction in the risk of disease progression for BCG (hazard ratio [HR] 0.73; $P = .001$).[32] Following supply shortages, production of TheraCys was discontinued; a competing strain of BCG vaccine (TICE; Merck) is now available.[33]

### PROVENGE

Sipuleucel-T (PROVENGE; Dendreon Corporation) was approved by the FDA in April 2010. PROVENGE is an autologous cellular immunotherapy indicated for the treatment of asymptomatic or minimally symptomatic mCRPC.[24] Autologous peripheral blood mononuclear cells, including APCs, are obtained via leukapheresis, then cultured with PA2024, the fusion product of the recombinant tumor antigen PAP and APC-activating GM-CSF. During a 40-h incubation, APCs process the recombinant antigen into peptides presented on their surface to effect MHC signaling and T-cell activation. Each dose of vaccine contains a minimum of 50 million autologous CD54+ (intercellular adhesion molecule 1 [ICAM-1])[34] cells activated with PAP-GM-CSF. Patients receive 3 doses given at 2-week intervals. The FDA initially rejected PROVENGE in 2007 after 2 phase III trials (D9901,[35] D9902A[36]) failed to meet their primary endpoints of progression-free survival (PFS). Analysis of the combined dataset demonstrated a 33% reduction in risk of death for PROVENGE ($P = .011$), leading to a third randomized phase III trial (D9902B, IMPACT)[37] with a primary endpoint of overall survival (OS) rather than PFS. Kantoff and colleagues demonstrated median OS of 25.8 months in the sipuleucel-T group versus 21.7 months in the placebo group, a 4.1-month benefit. There was a 22% relative reduction in risk of death with an HR of 0.78 (95% confidence interval [CI], 0.61–0.98; $P = .03$).

### IMLYGIC®

IMLYGIC (talimogene laherparepvec; Amgen), or T-VEC, is a genetically modified oncolytic viral therapy approved by the FDA in 2015 for the treatment of advanced melanoma.[38] Considered a type of therapeutic cancer vaccine, T-VEC represents a novel drug class using a genetically modified, live, attenuated herpesvirus that expresses GM-CSF. T-VEC has a dual mechanism of action, mediating both local and systemic immune responses. T-VEC is injected into unresectable cutaneous, subcutaneous, or nodal lesions in patients with recurrent melanoma, which produces a local tumoricidal effect through viral replication and cell lysis. GM-CSF produced during viral replication enhances T-cell priming by APCs that present tumor antigens released during viral-mediated tumor lysis. Tumor-antigen–loaded DCs migrate systemically and effect a distant immune response, although responses in injected tumor are superior to those of distant metastases.[39] After the initial treatment, subsequent doses of T-VEC can be administered at 3-week (dose 2) and 2-week (dose 3 and beyond) intervals for 6 months, or until no treatable lesions remain. FDA approval in 2015 followed a randomized, open-label, phase III trial (OPTiM, n = 436)[40] comparing intralesional T-VEC with subcutaneous GM-CSF. The primary endpoint of durable response rate (DRR) was defined as the percentage of patients with complete response or partial response maintained continuously for a minimum of 6 months. T-VEC resulted in both higher DRR and longer median OS. DRR in the T-VEC group was 16.3% versus 2.1% in the GM-CSF group ($P<.001$), with an overall response rate (ORR) of 26% versus 6%, respectively. Median OS was 23.3 months (95% CI, 19.5–29.6 months) with T-VEC and 18.9 months (95% CI, 16.0–23.7 months) with GM-CSF (HR 0.79; 95% CI, 0.62–1.00; $P = .051$).

## THERAPEUTIC VACCINE CLINICAL TRIALS
### Experience

Other than trials of BCG, sipuleucel-T, and T-VEC, phase III trials of cancer vaccine monotherapies have been largely negative (**Table 1**), despite these therapies being generally well tolerated with favorable side-effect profiles. Experience from these trials has shown that the kinetics of a clinical response to a therapeutic vaccine monotherapy are different from the kinetics of a response to cytotoxic chemotherapy, and that PFS is a poor proxy for clinical efficacy.[41] Fundamental differences between cytotoxic chemotherapy and cancer vaccine therapies account for the differing kinetics of response. Whereas chemotherapy attacks the tumor and its microenvironment, vaccines target the immune system itself. Chemotherapy can work quickly, but its tumoricidal properties are transient and limited by pharmacokinetics, drug half-life, and toxicity. In contrast, vaccines effect a delayed, memory immune response that may yield a distant survival benefit by precluding the spread and survival of micrometastatic disease.[42] The terms epitope spreading, antigen spreading, and antigen cascade all describe the broad T-cell response to non-vaccine tumor antigens that follows vaccine-mediated tumor lysis.[43] Antigen cascade may allow for the successful recognition and cross-priming of patient-specific tumor neoantigens, yielding a durable immune response that is more clinically meaningful than the initial response to the vaccine's targeted epitopes.[44] Both vaccine kinetics and clinical experience suggest that vaccine therapies are most effective in patients with good performance status, limited tumor burden, and slowly progressive, early-stage disease. Although complex immune endpoints resulting from antigen cascade are active targets of investigation, OS remains the best surrogate for clinical efficacy and the primary endpoint of most active vaccine trials.

### Current Strategies

As of October 2018, there are 522 active interventional studies of cancer vaccines (351 in the United States, 91 in Europe, and 50 in China) available for review on clinicaltrials. gov. Current trials seek to improve therapeutic vaccine efficacy either by targeting novel tumor antigens or employing vaccines in combination with other therapeutic

**Table 1**
**Selected negative phase III clinical trials of therapeutic cancer vaccines**

| Vaccine | Vaccine Platform | Patient Population | Trial | Year |
|---|---|---|---|---|
| PSA-TRICOM (PROSTVAC) | Recombinant viral (vaccinia and fowlpox) | mCRPC | PROSPECT[66] NCT01322490 | 2018 |
| recMAGE-A3 + AS15 (GSK 2132231A) | Protein (MAGE-A3 CT antigen) | Melanoma | DERMA[67] NCT00796445 | 2018 |
| Canvaxin + BCG | Allogeneic whole tumor cell | Melanoma | NCT00052156[68] | 2017 |
| Rindopepimut (CDX-110) | Peptide (EGFR) | Glioblastoma | ACT IV[69] NCT01480479 | 2017 |
| IMA901 | Peptide | RCC | IMPRINT[70] NCT01265901 | 2016 |
| Multiepitope peptide | Peptide (MART-1/gp 100/tyrosinase) | Melanoma | NCT01989572[71] | 2015 |
| Belagenpumatucel-L (Lucanix) | Allogeneic whole tumor cell | NSCLC | NCT00676507[72] | 2015 |
| Tecemotide (Stimuvax/L-BLP25) | Peptide (MUC1) | NSCLC | START[73] NCT00409188 | 2014 |
| Gp100 | Peptide (gp100) | Melanoma | NCT00094653[74] | 2010 |
| GVAX | Recombinant DNA (GM-CSF) | mCRPC | VITAL-1[75] & VITAL-2[76] NCT00089856 (terminated for futility) | 2008 |
| Bec2 + BCG | Ganglioside | SCLC | SILVA[77] NCT00003279 | 2008 |

*Abbreviations:* GVAX, GM-CSF–transduced autologous tumor-cell vaccine; NSCLC, non–small cell lung cancer; RCC, renal cell carcinoma; SCLC, small cell lung cancer.

approaches (**Fig. 1**). Combination strategies typically include chemotherapy, radiotherapy (RT), endocrine therapy, small-molecule inhibitors, cytokines, or immune checkpoint inhibitors (ICI). These therapies often exert secondary immune-mediated antineoplastic effects, and novel trials seek to exploit potential synergistic responses. For example, RT is an effective local anticancer therapy with known immune pathway synergies. Whereas the local tumoricidal effect of ionizing radiation is due to direct DNA damage and free radical production, RT has been shown to improve control of both locoregional and distant systemic disease. The abscopal effect (a term derived from the Latin words for "off target") was first described in 1953[45] following the observation that ionizing radiation slowed tumor growth outside of the radiation field. By 2004, the effect was shown to be immune mediated.[46] RT affects an immune response when tumor antigens are released from dying tumor cells and form an in situ vaccine.[47] RT monotherapy also generates maturation stimuli required for DC activation of T lymphocytes. RT upregulates the expression of MHC class I molecules, calreticulin, and high-mobility group box 1 (HMGB1) protein.[48] MHC class I is required to effect a T-cell–mediated response against tumor, and neoplastic cells often downregulate MHC expression as a means of immune evasion. Calreticulin is a calcium-binding chaperone that assists production of both MHC class I proteins and tapasin, a cofactor required for MHC assembly. Calreticulin promotes phagocytic uptake of TAAs, and an increase in calreticulin is associated with antitumor immunity.[49] HMGB1 is a highly conserved nuclear protein that acts as a proinflammatory cytokine

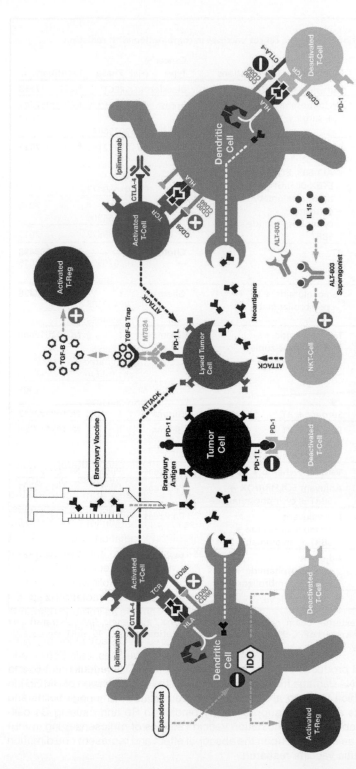

**Fig. 1.** Multimodal immunotherapy via multiple synergistic pathways can improve therapeutic vaccine efficacy. Vaccines targeting novel antigens (brachyury) generate antigen-specific T-cell–mediated response. Immune checkpoint inhibitors block PD-1, PD-L1, and CTLA-4 and inhibit immunosuppressive pathways that allow cancer cell evasion. TGF-β neutralization exerts a negative effect on activity of immunosuppressive Tregs and when combined with an ICI (M7824) enables T-cell infiltration of tumor. Stimulatory cytokines (ALT-803) enhance NK-cell–mediated cytotoxicity. Inhibition of the IDO enzyme (epacadostat) downregulates immunosuppressive pathways. Immunogenic tumor-cell death releases tumor neoantigens and increases downstream cross-priming of further T-cell response. (*Courtesy of* Z. Folzenlogen, MD, Denver, CO.)

**Table 2**
**Selected clinical trials of therapeutic cancer vaccines in combination with radiation**

| Vaccine | Combination Interventions | Cancer Type | Phase | Identifier |
|---|---|---|---|---|
| Intravesical BCG | Durvalumab + EBRT | Bladder | I/II | NCT03317158 |
| Autologous DC-adenovirus p53 vaccine | Cyclophosphamide + surgery + RT | Breast | I/II | NCT00082641 |
| Yeast-brachyury peptide vaccine (GI-6301) | Aldoxorubicin hydrochloride HCl, ALT-803, ETBX-051, ETBX-061, GI-6301, haNK, avelumab, cetuximab, cyclophosphamide, SBRT | Chordoma | I/II | NCT03647423 |
| Yeast-brachyury peptide vaccine (GI-6301) | RT | Chordoma | II | NCT02383498 |
| Personalized neoantigen vaccine (NeoVax) | Temozolomide + RT + pembrolizumab | Glioma | I | NCT02287428 |
| Autologous DCs pulsed with lysate derived from an allogeneic glioblastoma stem-like cell line | Temozolomide + RT ± bevacizumab | Glioma | I | NCT02010606 |
| HSPPC-96 | Surgery + RT | Glioma | I | NCT02722512 |
| HSPPC-96 | Surgery + RT + temozolomide + pembrolizumab | Glioma | II | NCT03018288 |
| GVAX | Vaccine + chemo + RT | Pancreas | Pilot | NCT00727441 |
| GVAX | Adjuvant FOLFIRINOX + SBRT + cyclophosphamide | Pancreas | Pilot | NCT01595321 |
| GVAX | Neoadjuvant cyclophosphamide + SBRT + nivolumab | Pancreas | II | NCT03161379 |
| GVAX | Adjuvant cyclophosphamide + SBRT + pembrolizumab | Pancreas | II | NCT02648282 |
| ProstAtak® (AdV-tk) | RT + valacyclovir | Prostate | III | NCT01436968 |

*Abbreviations:* EBRT, external beam radiation therapy; GVAX, allogeneic GM-CSF-transduced pancreatic tumor-cell vaccine; HSPPC-96, heat shock protein peptide complex-96; SBRT, stereotactic body radiation therapy.

stimulating the local production of tumor necrosis factor (TNF), interleukin (IL)-6, and interferon (IFN)-γ. DNA damage from radiation leads to the sequestration of HMGB1 in the cell nucleus, which leads to an increase in hypermutated immunoglobulins and DCs.[50] HMGB1 acts as a tumor suppressor by binding to Rb and causing G1 cell-cycle arrest and apoptosis.[51] Combination vaccine studies of radiosensitizing immunotherapy (**Table 2**) seek to build upon the abscopal effect and represent one direction of ongoing therapeutic vaccine research.

**Table 3**
**Cancer therapies with known immune synergies**

| Anticancer Therapy | Mechanism of Action to Enhance Vaccine Efficacy |
|---|---|
| Oxaliplatin<br>Anthracyclines | ↑ Release of tumor antigen following cell death<br>↑ Cross-priming of TAA by DC<br>↑ T-cell activation |
| Docetaxel | ↓ Tregs<br>Modulates CD4$^+$, CD8$^+$, CD19$^+$, NK (natural killer)<br>Enhances CD8$^+$ response to CD3 crosslinking |
| Paclitaxel | ↑ T-helper type I cytokine production patterns<br>(IFN-$\gamma$ and IL-2)<br>↑ CD44 in CD4$^+$ and CD8$^+$ effector T cells |
| Cisplatin<br>Vinorelbine | ↑ CD4$^+$ T cell: Treg |
| Cyclophosphamide | ↓ Treg function<br>↑ CD4$^+$ T-cell development<br>Modulates DC maturation and function |
| Fludarabine | ↓ Tregs |
| 5-FU | ↓ MDSC<br>↑ IFN-$\gamma$ production by intratumoral CD8$^+$ T cells |
| Temozolomide | Induces autophagy |
| Radiation therapy | ↑ Release of tumor antigen following cell death<br>(abscopal effect)<br>↑ Cross-priming of TAA by DC<br>↑ T-cell activation<br>↑ Calreticulin expression → ↑ MHC class I<br>↑ tapasin ↑ phagocytosis |
| Radionuclide therapy | ↑ Fas, CEA, MUC-1, MHC class I, ICAM-1 |
| Endocrine therapy | ↑ Thymic regeneration → ↑ naïve T cells |
| Sunitinib | ↓ Tregs ↓ MDSC<br>↑ Intratumoral infiltration of activated T lymphocytes |
| BCL-2 inhibitors | ↑ CD8$^+$ T cell: Treg |

Systemic standard-of-care anticancer therapies such as chemotherapy, endocrine therapies, and small-molecule–targeted agents may potentiate the antitumor effects of immunotherapy (as summarized in **Table 3**), and vice versa.[12] Many trials of ICIs have been negative, with approvals generally limited to hot tumors—those prone to immune recognition because of high mutational load and increased tumor neoantigen expression. Most tumors remain cold, however, unseen by the immune system. An unfavorable tumor microenvironment and low levels of circulating lymphocytes mean that ICIs are often ineffective. Novel combination strategies using therapeutic cancer vaccines offer the potential to turn cold tumors hot. Like RT, cytotoxic chemotherapy can induce immunogenic tumor-cell death through downstream cross-priming of released tumor antigens by APCs and T-cell activation. Chemotherapy can decrease populations of immunosuppressive regulatory T cells (Tregs)[52] or modulate their function. Small molecules such as sunitinib also decrease populations of Tregs and myeloid-derived suppressor cells (MDSC); BCL-2 inhibitors increase the ratio of CD8$^+$ cells to Tregs. Endocrine therapies can induce thymic regeneration, with increased numbers of naïve T cells. Like RT, systemic radionuclide therapies can upregulate expression of the Fas death receptor on tumor cells. Fas, or CD95, is a cell-surface protein that belongs to the TNF receptor family that mediates apoptosis and is often downregulated by cancer cells as a mechanism of immune evasion.[53] Therapeutic vaccine trials exploring immune synergies with standard-of-care therapies are ongoing.

Antigen cascade following therapeutic vaccination generates a population of tumor antigen-specific T cells. Most contemporary vaccine trials are investigating strategies of immunogenic intensification[54] through combined immune therapies that expand and facilitate this T-cell population while preventing immune tolerance and evasion. Phase I and II clinical trials exploring combinations of FDA-approved vaccines (sipuleucel-T, T-VEC) and FDA-approved ICIs (ipilimumab, pembrolizumab, nivolumab) have already demonstrated robust responses in combination arms.[55] Trials of vaccines in combination with antibodies to programmed cell death protein 1 (PD-1) and cytotoxic T-lymphocyte–associated protein 4 (CTLA-4) are generally more mature than those using FDA-approved antiprogrammed death ligand 1 (PD-L1) antibodies (avelumab, atezolizumab, durvalumab). Comprehensive reviews are available that detail these combined modality studies.[55,56] Novel non–FDA-approved vaccines are also finding success in combination with ICIs. An open-label phase II clinical trial (NCT02426892)[57] investigating a peptide vaccine (ISA101) targeting HPV oncoproteins E6 and E7 in patients with incurable HPV-16$^+$ solid tumors recently demonstrated that the addition of the vaccine to nivolumab generated an ORR of 33%, superior to that of single-agent anti-PD-1 antibodies previously tested in similar patient populations (CheckMate 141).[58]

Research from our group suggests that even deeper immunogenic intensification is possible through the concurrent use of multiple therapeutic classes. The National Cancer Institute's (NCI) intramural program has opened multidrug trials including QuEST1 (NCT03493945), a phase I/II trial of a brachyury-targeted vaccine in combination with M7824, ALT-803, and epacadostat. BN-Brachyury is a novel recombinant vector-based therapeutic cancer vaccine designed to induce an enhanced immune response against brachyury, which is overexpressed in many solid tumor types and is a transcription factor promoting epithelial-to-mesenchymal transition and metastatic spread.[15] M7824 is a bifunctional fusion protein consisting of an anti-PD-L1 antibody and the extracellular domain of transforming growth factor (TGF)-β receptor type 2, a TGF-β trap. TGF-β inhibits the immune response via multiple pathways, including expansion of Tregs,[59] and has been associated with metastatic progression.[60–62] M7824 can also mediate antibody-dependent cellular cytotoxicity (ADCC) in vitro. ALT-803 is an IL-15/IL-15Rα cytokine superagonist complex that can enhance natural killer cell–mediated ADCC and T-cell cytotoxicity.[63] Epacadostat (INCB024360) is an orally available inhibitor of indoleamine 2,3-dioxygenase, a tryptophan pathway enzyme overexpressed in many solid tumors that enhances immune escape.[64] Using a similar multimodality approach, NCT03050814 is a randomized phase II trial of a therapeutic vaccine (Ad-CEA) in combination with an anti-PD-L1 monoclonal antibody (avelumab) and standard-of-care chemotherapy (FOLFOX) for patients with metastatic colorectal cancer. Our group is also exploring intralesional versus systemic vaccine delivery as well as immunogenic intensification through novel combinations of multiple viral vectors and tumor antigens. NCT03481816 is a dose-escalation study of 3 separate adenovirus-vectored vaccines, each individually targeting the human TAAs PSA, MUC1, and brachyury. NCT03349983 is a dose-escalation study of 2 recombinant viral vectors (modified vaccinia Ankara and fowlpox) that express the T-cell costimulatory molecules B7.1, ICAM-1, and LFA-3 (designated TRICOM) and the tumor antigen brachyury.

Technological advances now allow for the processing of cold tumor into a personalized mutanome vaccine.[16] First-in-human trials of these vaccines compare biopsies of cold tumor and healthy tissue with next-generation sequencing assays that allow for the detection of tumor-specific neoantigens. Computational prediction algorithms then generate targets for neoepitope vaccines. Personalized mutanome vaccines have the potential for therapeutic benefit irrespective of tumor histology or intrinsic immunogenicity. The NCI's Surgery Branch has developed a pipeline to generate tumor neoantigens for personalized therapeutic vaccine trials. NCT03480152 is an open-label, phase I/II trial that identifies neoantigens following tumor resection and isolation of tumor-infiltrating lymphocytes (TILs). Immunogenic neoantigens will be identified from TILs by high-throughput immunologic screening using long peptides and tandem minigenes covering all mutated epitopes.[65] These neoantigens will form the basis of a therapeutic mRNA vaccine. A competing trial (NCT03300843) is using TILs to produce a personalized DC vaccine.

## SUMMARY

Cancer vaccines represent some of the most exciting developments in oncology in the last decade. Unfortunately, their impact as monotherapy in metastatic carcinomas has been modest. As of today, we have few positive clinical trials with 3 therapeutic cancer vaccines approved by the FDA. Many preclinical and clinical studies have suggested that therapeutic cancer vaccines can activate effector T cells against tumor antigens and kill targeted cells across different tumor types with minimal toxicities. Cancer vaccines also expand T-cell clones that can travel to disease sites, leading to increased tumor T-cell inflammation. Ideal additive and/or synergistic therapeutic agents in combination with cancer vaccines should be able to assist effector T cells by neutralizing local immunosuppressive mechanisms responsible for immune escape, with the ultimate goal of engaging, expanding, and enabling the antitumor immune response.

Future clinical trials will identify the timing and sequence of the best combination strategies. Important considerations in designing those trials include:

1. Adaptive design that can quickly detect the most effective combinations and eliminate nonactive ones
2. Detection and development of biomarkers of immune response
3. Optimal timing of treatment
4. Neoadjuvant studies that focus on the tumor microenvironment
5. Different vaccine platforms that can target the same antigens yet activate different T-cell populations
6. Analysis of local versus systemic vaccine delivery methods.

One of the major concerns of combination therapy has been the possibility of increased toxicity; however, data so far suggest that combinations do not result in any additional toxicity. Combinations of different treatment modalities such as chemotherapy, hormone therapy, radiopharmaceuticals, and ICIs with cancer vaccines have been proved safe in numerous trials. Results of ongoing and planned larger randomized studies will determine the future of immune-based treatment platforms.

## ACKNOWLEDGMENTS

The authors acknowledge the Intramural Research Program of the Center for Cancer Research, National Cancer Institute, National Institutes of Health, for its support in the production of this article. The authors also acknowledge the significant editing contributions of Bonnie L. Casey.

## REFERENCES

1. Galmarini D, Galmarini CM, Galmarini FC. Cancer chemotherapy: a critical analysis of its 60 years of history. Crit Rev Oncol Hematol 2012;84(2):181–99.
2. Coley WB. II. Contribution to the knowledge of sarcoma. Ann Surg 1891;14(3): 199–220.
3. Coley WB. The treatment of malignant tumors by repeated inoculations of erysipelas. With a report of ten original cases. Clin Orthop Relat Res 1893;1991(262): 3–11.
4. Coley WB. Treatment of inoperable malignant tumors with toxins of erysipelas and the Bacillus prodigiosus. Trans Am Surg Assoc 1894;12:183–212.
5. Coley WB. The treatment of inoperable sarcoma by bacterial toxins (the mixed toxins of the *Streptococcus erysipelas* and the *Bacillus prodigiosus*). Proc R Soc Med 1910;3(Surg Sect):1–48.
6. Johnston BJ, Novales ET. Clinical effect of Coley's toxin. II. A seven-year study. Cancer Chemother Rep 1962;21:43–68.
7. Barquet N, Domingo P. Smallpox: the triumph over the most terrible of the ministers of death. Ann Intern Med 1997;127(8 Pt 1):635–42.
8. Jenner E. An inquiry into the causes and effects of the variolae vaccinae, a disease discovered in some of the western counties of England, particularly Gloucestershire, and known by the name of the cow pox. London: Sampson Low; 1798.
9. Arita I, Breman JG. Evaluation of smallpox vaccination policy. Bull World Health Organ 1979;57(1):1–9.
10. Lollini PL, Cavallo F, Nanni P, et al. Vaccines for tumour prevention. Nat Rev Cancer 2006;6(3):204–16.
11. Herlyn D, Birebent B. Advances in cancer vaccine development. Ann Med 1999; 31(1):66–78.
12. Schlom J, Hodge JW, Palena C, et al. Therapeutic cancer vaccines. Adv Cancer Res 2014;121:67–124.
13. Gjerstorff MF, Andersen MH, Ditzel HJ. Oncogenic cancer/testis antigens: prime candidates for immunotherapy. Oncotarget 2015;6(18):15772–87.
14. Xiang R, Luo Y, Niethammer AG, et al. Oral DNA vaccines target the tumor vasculature and microenvironment and suppress tumor growth and metastasis. Immunol Rev 2008;222:117–28.
15. Fernando RI, Litzinger M, Trono P, et al. The T-box transcription factor Brachyury promotes epithelial-mesenchymal transition in human tumor cells. J Clin Invest 2010;120(2):533–44.
16. Sahin U, Tureci O. Personalized vaccines for cancer immunotherapy. Science 2018;359(6382):1355–60.
17. Hou Y, Kavanagh B, Fong L. Distinct CD8+ T cell repertoires primed with agonist and native peptides derived from a tumor-associated antigen. J Immunol 2008; 180(3):1526–34.
18. Parmiani G, Pilla L, Maccalli C, et al. Autologous versus allogeneic cell-based vaccines? Cancer J 2011;17(5):331–6.
19. Hanna MG Jr, Peters LC. Specific immunotherapy of established visceral micrometastases by BCG-tumor cell vaccine alone or as an adjunct to surgery. Cancer 1978;42(6):2613–25.
20. Berger M, Kreutz FT, Horst JL, et al. Phase I study with an autologous tumor cell vaccine for locally advanced or metastatic prostate cancer. J Pharm Pharm Sci 2007;10(2):144–52.

21. Guo C, Manjili MH, Subjeck JR, et al. Therapeutic cancer vaccines: past, present, and future. Adv Cancer Res 2013;119:421–75.

22. Sondak VK, Sabel MS, Mule JJ. Allogeneic and autologous melanoma vaccines: where have we been and where are we going? Clin Cancer Res 2006;12(7 Pt 2): 2337s–41s.

23. Banchereau J, Steinman RM. Dendritic cells and the control of immunity. Nature 1998;392(6673):245–52.

24. FDA. PROVENGE: highlights of prescribing information. Available at: https://www.fda.gov/downloads/biologicsbloodvaccines/cellulargenetherapyproducts/approvedproducts/UCM210031.pdf. Accessed September 1, 2018.

25. Bitton RJ, Guthmann MD, Gabri MR, et al. Cancer vaccines: an update with special focus on ganglioside antigens. Oncol Rep 2002;9(2):267–76.

26. FDA. UNITUXIN: highlights of prescribing information. Available at: https://www.accessdata.fda.gov/drugsatfda_docs/label/2015/125516s000lbl.pdf. Accessed September 1, 2018.

27. Morton D, Ravindranath M, Irie R. Tumor gangliosides as targets for active specific immunotherapies of melanoma in man. In: Svennerholm L, Asbury A, Reisfeld R, editors. Progress in brain research. Amsterdam: Elsevier; 1994. p. 251–75.

28. Kirkwood JM, Ibrahim JG, Sosman JA, et al. High-dose interferon alfa-2b significantly prolongs relapse-free and overall survival compared with the GM2-KLH/QS-21 vaccine in patients with resected stage IIB-III melanoma: results of intergroup trial E1694/S9512/C509801. J Clin Oncol 2001;19(9):2370–80.

29. Yang B, Jeang J, Yang A, et al. DNA vaccine for cancer immunotherapy. Hum Vaccin Immunother 2014;10(11):3153–64.

30. Sanofi. TheraCys: highlights of prescribing information. Available at: https://www.vaccineshoppe.com/image.cfm?doc_id=12635&image_type=product_pdf. Accessed September 1, 2018.

31. Lamm DL, Blumenstein BA, Crawford ED, et al. A randomized trial of intravesical doxorubicin and immunotherapy with bacille Calmette-Guerin for transitional-cell carcinoma of the bladder. N Engl J Med 1991;325(17):1205–9.

32. Sylvester RJ, van der MA, Lamm DL. Intravesical bacillus Calmette-Guerin reduces the risk of progression in patients with superficial bladder cancer: a meta-analysis of the published results of randomized clinical trials. J Urol 2002; 168(5):1964–70.

33. FDA. TICE BCG: prescribing information. Available at: https://www.fda.gov/downloads/biologicsbloodvaccines/vaccines/approvedproducts/ucm163039.pdf. Accessed September 1, 2018.

34. Sheikh NA, Jones LA. CD54 is a surrogate marker of antigen presenting cell activation. Cancer Immunol Immunother 2008;57(9):1381–90.

35. Small EJ, Schellhammer PF, Higano CS, et al. Placebo-controlled phase III trial of immunologic therapy with sipuleucel-T (APC8015) in patients with metastatic, asymptomatic hormone refractory prostate cancer. J Clin Oncol 2006;24(19): 3089–94.

36. Higano CS, Schellhammer PF, Small EJ, et al. Integrated data from 2 randomized, double-blind, placebo-controlled, phase 3 trials of active cellular immunotherapy with sipuleucel-T in advanced prostate cancer. Cancer 2009;115(16):3670–9.

37. Kantoff PW, Higano CS, Shore ND, et al. Sipuleucel-T immunotherapy for castration-resistant prostate cancer. N Engl J Med 2010;363(5):411–22.

38. FDA. IMLYGIC: Highlights of prescribing information. Available at: https://www.fda.gov/downloads/BiologicsBloodVaccines/CellularGeneTherapyProducts/ApprovedProducts/UCM469575.pdf. Accessed September 1, 2018.
39. Conry RM, Westbrook B, McKee S, et al. Talimogene laherparepvec: first in class oncolytic virotherapy. Hum Vaccin Immunother 2018;14(4):839–46.
40. Andtbacka RH, Kaufman HL, Collichio F, et al. Talimogene laherparepvec improves durable response rate in patients with advanced melanoma. J Clin Oncol 2015;33(25):2780–8.
41. Gulley JL, Madan RA, Heery CR. Therapeutic vaccines and immunotherapy in castration-resistant prostate cancer: current progress and clinical applications. Am Soc Clin Oncol Educ Book 2013. https://doi.org/10.1200/EdBook_AM.2013.33.e166.
42. Stein WD, Gulley JL, Schlom J, et al. Tumor regression and growth rates determined in five intramural NCI prostate cancer trials: the growth rate constant as an indicator of therapeutic efficacy. Clin Cancer Res 2011;17(4):907–17.
43. Gulley JL, Madan RA, Tsang KY, et al. Immune impact induced by PROSTVAC (PSA-TRICOM), a therapeutic vaccine for prostate cancer. Cancer Immunol Res 2014;2(2):133–41.
44. Hardwick N, Chain B. Epitope spreading contributes to effective immunotherapy in metastatic melanoma patients. Immunotherapy 2011;3(6):731–3.
45. Mole RH. Whole body irradiation; radiobiology or medicine? Br J Radiol 1953;26(305):234–41.
46. Demaria S, Ng B, Devitt ML, et al. Ionizing radiation inhibition of distant untreated tumors (abscopal effect) is immune mediated. Int J Radiat Oncol Biol Phys 2004;58(3):862–70.
47. Grass GD, Krishna N, Kim S. The immune mechanisms of abscopal effect in radiation therapy. Curr Probl Cancer 2016;40(1):10–24.
48. Sharabi AB, Lim M, DeWeese TL, et al. Radiation and checkpoint blockade immunotherapy: radiosensitisation and potential mechanisms of synergy. Lancet Oncol 2015;16(13):e498–509.
49. Raghavan M, Wijeyesakere SJ, Peters LR, et al. Calreticulin in the immune system: ins and outs. Trends Immunol 2013;34(1):13–21.
50. Martinotti S, Patrone M, Ranzato E. Emerging roles for HMGB1 protein in immunity, inflammation, and cancer. Immunotargets Ther 2015;4:101–9.
51. Jiao Y, Wang HC, Fan SJ. Growth suppression and radiosensitivity increase by HMGB1 in breast cancer. Acta Pharmacol Sin 2007;28(12):1957–67.
52. Roselli M, Cereda V, di Bari MG, et al. Effects of conventional therapeutic interventions on the number and function of regulatory T cells. Oncoimmunology 2013;2(10):e27025.
53. Peter ME, Hadji A, Murmann AE, et al. The role of CD95 and CD95 ligand in cancer. Cell Death Differ 2015;22(4):549–59.
54. O'Sullivan Coyne G, Gulley JL. Adding fuel to the fire: immunogenic intensification. Hum Vaccin Immunother 2014;10(11):3306–12.
55. Collins JM, Redman JM, Gulley JL. Combining vaccines and immune checkpoint inhibitors to prime, expand, and facilitate effective tumor immunotherapy. Expert Rev Vaccines 2018;17(8):697–705.
56. Gatti-Mays ME, Redman JM, Collins JM, et al. Cancer vaccines: enhanced immunogenic modulation through therapeutic combinations. Hum Vaccin Immunother 2017;13(11):2561–74.
57. Massarelli E, William W, Johnson F, et al. Combining immune checkpoint blockade and tumor-specific vaccine for patients with incurable human

papillomavirus 16-related cancer: a phase 2 clinical trial. JAMA Oncol 2018. [Epub ahead of print]. https://doi.org/10.1001/jamaoncol.2018.4051.

58. Ferris RL, Blumenschein G Jr, Fayette J, et al. Nivolumab vs investigator's choice in recurrent or metastatic squamous cell carcinoma of the head and neck: 2-year long-term survival update of CheckMate 141 with analyses by tumor PD-L1 expression. Oral Oncol 2018;81:45–51.

59. Kanamori M, Nakatsukasa H, Okada M, et al. Induced regulatory T cells: their development, stability, and applications. Trends Immunol 2016;37(11):803–11.

60. Larocca C, Cohen JR, Fernando RI, et al. An autocrine loop between TGF-beta1 and the transcription factor brachyury controls the transition of human carcinoma cells into a mesenchymal phenotype. Mol Cancer Ther 2013;12(9):1805–15.

61. Jakowlew SB. Transforming growth factor-beta in cancer and metastasis. Cancer Metastasis Rev 2006;25(3):435–57.

62. Derynck R, Akhurst RJ, Balmain A. TGF-beta signaling in tumor suppression and cancer progression. Nat Genet 2001;29(2):117–29.

63. Robinson TO, Schluns KS. The potential and promise of IL-15 in immuno-oncogenic therapies. Immunol Lett 2017;190:159–68.

64. Holmgaard RB, Zamarin D, Munn DH, et al. Indoleamine 2,3-dioxygenase is a critical resistance mechanism in antitumor T cell immunotherapy targeting CTLA-4. J Exp Med 2013;210(7):1389–402.

65. Lu YC, Yao X, Crystal JS, et al. Efficient identification of mutated cancer antigens recognized by T cells associated with durable tumor regressions. Clin Cancer Res 2014;20(13):3401–10.

66. Gulley JL, Borre M, Vogelzang N, et al. Results of PROSPECT: a randomized phase 3 trial of PROSTVAC-V/F (PRO) in men with asymptomatic or minimally symptomatic metastatic, castration-resistant prostate cancer. J Clin Oncol 2018;36(15 suppl) [abstract: 5006].

67. Dreno B, Thompson JF, Smithers BM, et al. MAGE-A3 immunotherapeutic as adjuvant therapy for patients with resected, MAGE-A3-positive, stage III melanoma (DERMA): a double-blind, randomised, placebo-controlled, phase 3 trial. Lancet Oncol 2018;19(7):916–29.

68. Faries MB, Mozzillo N, Kashani-Sabet M, et al. Long-term survival after complete surgical resection and adjuvant immunotherapy for distant melanoma metastases. Ann Surg Oncol 2017;24(13):3991–4000.

69. Weller M, Butowski N, Tran DD, et al. Rindopepimut with temozolomide for patients with newly diagnosed, EGFRvIII-expressing glioblastoma (ACT IV): a randomised, double-blind, international phase 3 trial. Lancet Oncol 2017;18(10): 1373–85.

70. Rini BI, Stenzl A, Zdrojowy R, et al. IMA901, a multipeptide cancer vaccine, plus sunitinib versus sunitinib alone, as first-line therapy for advanced or metastatic renal cell carcinoma (IMPRINT): a multicentre, open-label, randomised, controlled, phase 3 trial. Lancet Oncol 2016;17(11):1599–611.

71. Lawson DH, Lee S, Zhao F, et al. Randomized, placebo-controlled, phase III trial of yeast-derived granulocyte-macrophage colony-stimulating factor (GM-CSF) versus peptide vaccination versus GM-CSF plus peptide vaccination versus placebo in patients with no evidence of disease after complete surgical resection of locally advanced and/or stage IV melanoma: a trial of the Eastern Cooperative Oncology Group-American College of Radiology Imaging Network Cancer Research Group (E4697). J Clin Oncol 2015;33(34):4066–76.

72. Giaccone G, Bazhenova LA, Nemunaitis J, et al. A phase III study of belagenpumatucel-L, an allogeneic tumour cell vaccine, as maintenance therapy for non-small cell lung cancer. Eur J Cancer 2015;51(16):2321–9.
73. Butts C, Socinski MA, Mitchell PL, et al. Tecemotide (L-BLP25) versus placebo after chemoradiotherapy for stage III non-small-cell lung cancer (START): a randomised, double-blind, phase 3 trial. Lancet Oncol 2014;15(1):59–68.
74. Hodi FS, O'Day SJ, McDermott DF, et al. Improved survival with ipilimumab in patients with metastatic melanoma. N Engl J Med 2010;363(8):711–23.
75. Cell genesys announces termination of VITAL-1 phase 3 clinical trial of GVAX immunotherapy for prostate cancer based on outcome of futility analysis and reports preliminary analysis of VITAL-2 trial results. Available at: https://www.businesswire.com/news/home/20081016005394/en/Cell-Genesys-Announces-Termination-VITAL-1-Phase-3. Accessed September 1, 2018.
76. Cell genesys halts VITAL-2 GVAX trial in advanced prostate cancer. Available at: https://malecare.org/cell-genesys-halts-vital-2-gvax-trial-in-advanced-prostate-cancer/. Accessed September 1, 2018.
77. Bottomley A, Debruyne C, Felip E, et al. Symptom and quality of life results of an international randomised phase III study of adjuvant vaccination with Bec2/BCG in responding patients with limited disease small-cell lung cancer. Eur J Cancer 2008;44(15):2178–84.

# Innate Immune Stimulation in Cancer Therapy

Peter Düwell, PhD[a,1], Simon Heidegger, MD[b,1], Sebastian Kobold, MD[c,1,*]

## KEYWORDS

- Oncoimmunology • Innate immunity • NLR • TLR • STING • RLH • Antibodies
- Cancer

## KEY POINTS

- Imiquimod is the only TLR agonist currently approved for cancer therapy (for topical use).
- Mifamurtide is the only NOD agonist approved for adjuvant cancer therapy (osteosarcoma).
- STING, RIG-I, and NLRP3 agonists are in clinical testing.
- Strategies to directly target NK cells for cancer treatment are under clinical investigation.
- Innate immunity-based strategies are promising and might enhance combination therapies.

## INTRODUCTION

Arming the immune system to fight malignancies is predominantly based on (re-)activating the host's immune system to recognize and eliminate abnormally transformed cells. From an immunologic perspective, tumors can be classified into "hot" tumors, which show high infiltration by T cells and other immune cells, as opposed to "cold" tumors lacking those components. In principle, both categories can contain specific T cells, although they may lack functionality and display an exhausted phenotype.[1,2] Strategies to overcome these resistance mechanisms have so far included the use of antibodies directed at T cell–suppressive immune checkpoint molecules such as PD-1 (pembrolizumab and nivolumab), PD-L1 (atezolizumab; avelumab, and durvalumab), and CTLA-4 (ipilimumab).[3–5] Another strategy is the therapeutic use of T cells, so-called adoptive cell therapy.[6–10] Although these strategies are now established

Disclosure Statement: No disclosures from either author.
[a] Institute of Innate Immunity, University of Bonn, Sigmund-Freud-Strasse 25, 53127 Bonn, Germany; [b] Medizinische Klinik und Poliklinik 3, Klinikum rechts der Isar, Technische Universität München, Ismaningerstrasse 22, Munich 81675, Germany; [c] Division of Clinical Pharmacology, Center of Integrated Protein Science Munich (CIPS-M), Klinikum der Universität München, Lindwurmstrasse 2a, Munich 80337, Germany
[1] Authors contributed equally.
* Corresponding author. Lindwurmstrasse 2a, Munich 80337, Germany
E-mail address: sebastian.kobold@med.uni-muenchen.de

and their role in today's cancer care is expanding, it has become clear that most patients do not benefit over the long term, necessitating additional and innovative approaches.

One promising approach is the combination of the aforementioned therapies with chemo- and radiotherapy to enhance antitumor responses (reviewed by Yan and colleagues[11]). An interesting aspect of both chemotherapy and radiotherapy is that their immune-modulatory functions are based on triggering innate immune-recognition pathways. These receptors sense endogenous danger-associated molecular patterns (DAMPs), for example, cytosolic DNA, ATP, and alarmins (eg, cytokines), which are released on cell death, and exogenous pathogen-associated molecular patterns (PAMPs), which might lead to cell death (reviewed by Zitvogel and colleagues[12]). Both DAMPs and PAMPs are sensed by pattern-recognition receptors (PRR), which comprise a heterogenous family of germline-encoded innate immune receptors.[13] PRRs include nucleic acid-sensing receptors such as cGAS/STING, RIG-I-like helicases (RLHs), toll-like receptors (TLRs), and the large family of nucleotide-binding oligomerization domain (NOD)-like receptors (NLRs) with the most prominent members NOD2 and NLRP3. Although most of these receptors are expressed by various cells and tissues, it is predominantly the myeloid cell compartment that forms the first line of defense against invading pathogens.

Cancer is frequently associated with chronic inflammation, which is often considered a requirement for maintaining an immunosuppressive tumor network. Thus, triggering PRRs might seem counteractive as it would result in the secretion of proinflammatory cytokines and thereby further support chronic inflammation. However, PRR signaling also leads to cell activation with enhanced phagocytosis and increased expression of human leukocyte antigen (HLA) molecules (MHC-I). For example, pattern recognition by RLH ligands leads to upregulation of MHC-I molecules on tumor cells and type I interferon (IFN) secretion. This, in turn, enhances the presentation of tumor-related antigens and the induction of immunogenic cell death, which again unmasks tumors toward recognition and eradication by the immune system.[14] Another interesting set of innate receptors identified on natural killer (NK) cells are the killer cell immunoglobulin-like receptors (KIRs), which can distinguish malignant from healthy cells on the basis of peptides loaded on MHC molecules.[15,16]

More than a century ago, William Coley injected live or attenuated bacteria and pioneered tumor immunotherapy. Today, our current understanding of tumor immunology has recognized that PRR are of great importance to antitumor immunity.[17] Thus, the quality of initiating an innate immune response constitutes a critical prerequisite for linking innate and adaptive immunity. Here, the authors summarize advances in innate cancer immunotherapy by discussing the most important receptor families of the innate immune system and their implementation in effective therapy. The authors focus on present approaches and provide a future perspective of promising strategies that have the potency to complement the current repertoire of anticancer treatments (**Fig. 1**).

## TOLL-LIKE RECEPTOR AGONISTS

TLRs encompass a family of PRRs initially identified in the fruit fly.[18] TLRs sense different molecular patterns of microorganisms (bacterial, viral, and fungal), which results in the initiation of innate immune responses.[19,20] In humans, 10 different TLRs have been identified so far that serve as a first line of defense against invading pathogens.[18] TLRs can be roughly subdivided into endosomal and membrane-bound TLR.s Endosomal TLR3, 7, 8, and 9 sense intracellular patterns, particularly nucleic

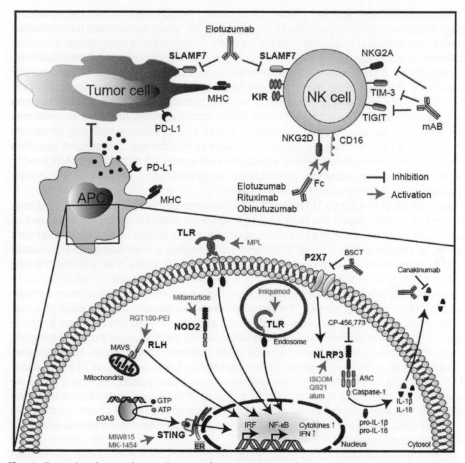

**Fig. 1.** Targeting innate immunity to achieve antitumor immunity. NK cells and antigen-presenting cells (APC) play a major role in tumor-directed immune responses. Monoclonal antibodies (mAB), such as elotuzumab, target inhibitory surface receptors and enhance NK-cell cytotoxic functions. Other mAB-targeting inhibitory signaling pathways (NKG2A, TIM-3, TIGIT) are being evaluated. In addition, FcγRIII- or NKG2D-mediated cytotoxicity by mAB-Fc portions have been described.[115,125] Membrane-bound TLRs can be specifically activated (monophosphoryl lipid A [MPL]; imiquimod) to elicit a predominantly NF-κB–driven proinflammatory immune response. Cytosolic receptors, such as nucleic acid-sensing cGAS/STING and RIG-I–like helicases (RLH), are activated by RNA (RGT100-PEI) or small-molecule compounds (MIW815; MK-1454) and lead to type I IFN as well as other interferon regulatory factor (IRF)-transcribed genes. NOD2, a cytosolic receptor for bacterial cell-wall components (mifamurtide), activates NF-κB–mediated gene transcription. The NLRP3 inflammasome can be activated by the ionotropic transmembrane receptor P2X7 and diverse stimuli (ISCOM, QS21, alum) that lead to activated caspase-1 and subsequent secretion of IL-1β and IL-18. Targeting P2X7 (BSCT) or NLRP3 (CP-456,773) prevents the release of IL-1 family cytokines. Canakinumab is an mAB specifically targeting IL-1β. ER, endoplasmatic reticulum.

acids. Membrane-bound TLR, such as TLR1, 2, 4, 5, 6, and 10, detect a plethora of microbial patterns including cell-wall components and lipopolysaccharides (LPS).[18] On activation, TLRs induce a proinflammatory response that contributes to pathogen clearance.[20] The potency of TLR agonists has been recognized early; only traces of the endotoxin LPS are sufficient to induce massive immune activation.[21]

The most ancient reported use of TLR agonists, though unknown at that time, date back to Coley's case series in the nineteenth century, when he reported cancer remission on intralesional challenge with live bacteria.[22] Thereafter it took almost a century before the first bacterial components were approved for clinical use: Bacille Calmette Guérin (BCG), an attenuated form of *Mycobacterium bovis*, is approved for intravesical treatment of localized urothelial carcinoma of the bladder in an adjuvant setting.[23] Currently BCG-mediated TLR signaling, with subsequent immune cell activation and recruitment, is proposed to be central for its activity. Although these experiences have invigorated research and clinical exploration of TLR immune signaling for cancer treatment, it rapidly became clear that broad expression and consequent toxicities resulting from excessive immune activation limit systemic application of TLR agonists.[23,24] As a consequence, many clinical programs using different TLR agonists, including the TLR9 agonist CpG, have failed.[25]

As of 2018, only a single TLR agonist has been approved as monotherapy for cancer treatment in topical use: the RNA analog imiquimod is approved for the treatment of basal cell carcinoma and precancerous lesions such as actinic keratosis.[24] Imiquimod binds to endosomal TLR7 and TLR8 and thus initiates a proinflammatory cascade, which culminates in a type I IFN response and requires the adapter protein MyD88.[19] In addition, imiquimod has also been shown to activate the NLRP3 inflammasome.[26] Applied topically, imiquimod induces complete remission in most patients treated, often avoiding surgery. Though deemed exceptionally safe in topical use, imiquimod comes with severe side effects when applied systemically because it rapidly blocks mitochondrial complex I, leading to enhanced inflammation-induced toxicity.[26] Thus, its development for systemic application has been discontinued. However, imiquimod is still under investigation for the treatment of skin metastases or in combination regimens.[27] Numerous TLR agonists have been tested as stand-alone or combination treatment in several tumor types over the years. Antitumor activity has been disappointing so far, being associated with severe toxicities or not reproducible in larger trials. Several excellent reviews give a good overview of the clinical trial landscape in recent years.[23,28–30]

A different application for TLR agonists in cancer immunotherapy is their use as vaccine adjuvants, applied locally to boost immune responses against the vaccine antigen. Whereas therapeutic vaccination against cancer has been controversial and remains to be proved in larger prospective trials, preventive vaccination (particularly in virally induced cancers) has already proved exceptional efficacy.[31] So far, only a TLR4 agonist, monophosphoryl lipid A (MPL), has gained approval as adjuvant to a human papilloma virus (HPV) vaccine to prevent infection and, subsequently, HPV-driven cervical cancer in young women.[23] Such vaccines are now part of the recommended preventive vaccination schedules in many countries. Although MPL has not been compared in larger clinical trials with other adjuvants in the same indication, these data demonstrate the potency of TLR agonists in vaccine development. An elegant strategy might be the combination of vaccine and adjuvant in a single molecule, as seen in ongoing efforts to use mRNA vaccines.[32] Hereby, the mRNA (1) encodes the target vaccine protein and (2) serves as a TLR7 agonist to activate innate and adaptive immunity. Ongoing and future research will demonstrate whether TLR agonists or other adjuvants might contribute to cancer treatment in a vaccine setting.

## NOD-LIKE RECEPTORS AND INFLAMMASOMES

Despite their critical function in the recognition and elimination of pathogens, PRRs play an important role in preserving tissue homeostasis, wound healing, and resolution of inflammatory processes on tissue damage.[33,34] The NLRs comprise a heterogenous family of cytosolic receptors.[35] Activation mechanisms of NLR are still a matter of debate, and specific activating ligands are only known for a few members so far. Mechanistically, the NOD domain contains ATP-GTPase-specific motifs, whereas the leucine-rich repeat is involved in ligand binding or sensing. The N-terminal domain is of importance because it determines downstream signaling through the interaction with other proteins, such as pyrin domain (PYD)-containing and caspase activation and recruitment domain (CARD)-containing proteins. Activation of NLR proteins results in the activation of the transcription factor nuclear factor κB (NF-κB) or effector caspases that further lead to the secretion of proinflammatory cytokines.

Within the preclinical realm, a plethora of agonists and antagonists have been developed but only a few compounds have entered clinical trials. The NLR CARD proteins NOD1 (NLRC1) and NOD2 (NLRC2) recognize bacterial cell-wall components from gram-positive as well as gram-negative bacteria.[36,37] Mifamurtide, a liposomal-formulated fully synthetic muramyl dipeptide, is the only compound binding NOD2 with clinical approval, for the adjuvant treatment of localized osteosarcoma following surgical resection. In contrast to NOD1, which is expressed in both the hematopoietic and nonhematopoietic compartment, NOD2 is mostly restricted to the hematopoietic compartment and certain epithelial cells within the small intestine.[38] Defects in both *NOD* genes have been shown to increase the susceptibility to colorectal cancer in preclinical murine models,[39,40] and are associated with *Helicobacter pylori*-related gastric cancers in humans.[41] Besides gastrointestinal tumors, involvement of NOD1/2 has also been associated with other cancers such as breast, prostate, ovarian, and lung carcinomas.[42,43] The aforementioned studies suggest that NOD1/2 can be considered as gatekeepers that not only preserve intestinal immune homeostasis by controlling bacterial homeostasis, but also control cancer development. Thus, NOD1 and NOD2 are attractive candidates for further evaluation in tumor immunotherapy.

Most NLR proteins form inflammasomes, involving the adapter molecule apoptosis-associated speck-like protein containing a CARD (ASC) and caspase-1 for effector function.[44] Activation of inflammasomes leads to proteolytic cleavage of procaspase-1 and subsequent activation of pro-interleukin (IL)-1β and pro-IL-18 into their active and secreted forms.[45] Activation of inflammasomes, however, is tightly regulated and requires a two-step mechanism: (1) transcriptional priming of the NLR protein and the proforms of IL-1β and IL-18; and (2) an activation step for inflammasome assembly, caspase-1–mediated cleavage of IL-1β/IL-18, and pyroptotic cell death.[45,46] Inflammasome members have been shown to be involved in cancer development, and coding variants of NLR have been associated with an increased risk for different cancer types.[47–53] The CARD domain–containing NLRC4 and the PYD domain–containing NLRP3 inflammasome are the best characterized NLR members, but direct ligands, so far, have only been identified for NLRC4.[54] Compared with TLR ligands, where clinical trials are available (see TLR section) no inflammasome activators are currently under investigation for their use in human patients.[45]

NLRP3 is the most-studied inflammasome member, and its contribution to diseases is controversial. NRLP3 is a sensor of cellular and metabolic stress, which is reflected by its activation mechanisms including lysosomal damage by crystalline structures such as β-amyloid (Alzheimer's disease), cholesterol crystals (atherosclerosis), and uric acid (gout),[55–57] stress-induced oxidized mitochondrial DNA and reactive oxygen species,[58,59] and lowering of potassium concentrations by pore-forming toxins or membrane channels.[60,61] NLRP3 acts as a central hub by condensing all this information into downstream IL-1β and IL-18 signaling. IL-1β has pleiotropic effects and, besides its role in inflammatory diseases, has been shown to have a tumor-promoting role in many cancers including melanoma, gastric cancer, and skin cancer.[62-64] Unlike IL-1β, IL-18 seems to exert protection and is important for epithelial damage repair.[65] Because IL-18 is an important inducer of IFN-γ, it is required for optimal priming of adaptive immune responses. Consequently, a phase II clinical trial showed that recombinant IL-18 was sufficient to induce antitumor effects, although it failed as a single-agent treatment in patients with metastatic melanoma.[66] Thus, a promising strategy might be the direct targeting of downstream cytokines rather than inflammasomes themselves. This is supported by the CANTOS trial, which was designed to assess the efficacy of the US Food and Drug Administration–approved monoclonal antibody canakinumab targeting IL-1β in patients with cardiovascular disease.[67] Intriguingly, meta-analysis of the trial suggested that long-term blocking of IL-1β with canakinumab could significantly reduce lung cancer incidence and mortality.[68] Further investigations are necessary to confirm current data and to test the possibility of blocking IL-1β in other cancer entities. At present, 3 clinical trials are testing canakinumab in the treatment of non–small cell lung cancer (NCT03447769; NCT03631199; NCT03626545).

Emerging evidence further suggests that activating inflammasome signaling might serve as an immune adjuvant for effective tumor therapy. Targeting upstream NLRP3 activation is difficult, as druggable targets are sparse. An upstream receptor known to activate NLRP3 is the purine receptor P2X7, which also senses high concentrations of extracellular ATP released from dying cells.[69,70] A phase I study is investigating the safety and tolerability of a BSCT (Anti-nf-P2X7) 10% ointment in patients with basal cell carcinoma (NCT02587819), and another study is investigating P2X7 as biomarker for uterine and endothelial cancer (NCT00471120). Of note, the TLR7 agonist imiquimod was recently shown to activate NLRP3, indicating that NLRP3 might also contribute to its anticancer effects.[26] Adjuvant potential of NLRP3 activation to boost adaptive immunity has already been shown for other compounds in the setting of tumor vaccination. The vaccine adjuvants QS21 (a saponin-based compound) and alum (aluminum hydroxide) are known to be potent NLRP3 activators.[71,72] However, aluminum's potential as an adjuvant remains controversial.[73] ISCOM (immune stimulating complex; cage-like structures consisting of saponin, phospholipids, and cholesterol[74]) are prophylactic as well as therapeutic vaccine adjuvants, and potent activators of the NLRP3 inflammasome.[75-77] ISCOM can be formulated with tumor antigen for effective cross-presentation and immune activation.[75-78] In preclinical models, ISCOM formulated with NY-ESO1, a cancer testis antigen, has also been found to be effective and to confer protection in a prophylactic setting against melanoma.[79,80] ISCOM formulations are considered safe[81] and have been tested for efficacy in different tumor entities, so far with limited success (NCT00518206; NCT00199901; NCT00851643; NCT02054104; NCT01341496; NCT01258868).

Finally, the NLRP3 antagonist CP-456,773 (also known as Cytokine Release Inhibitory Drug 3, CRID3, or MCC950) has shown promising effects in inflammatory diseases and cancer,[82,83] and clinical studies are expected soon. Of note, an agonistic NLRP3 compound is also planned to enter phase I clinical trials in 2018.[84] It is important to consider that targeting such a central hub might be problematic because inhibition could increase the risk of severe infection and activation could lead to enhanced autoinflammation. While we are awaiting the efficacy of NLRP3-specific compounds in clinical investigations, preclinical data already favor this approach for cancer immunotherapy.

## STING AGONISTS

For a long time it remained nebulous as to how antigen-presenting cells (APCs) can effectively cross-present tumor-associated antigens to T cells in the absence of microbial DAMPs, and thus, costimulation. It became clear that PRRs can, under certain conditions, detect endogenous molecular patterns, resulting in sterile inflammation.[85] Recently, tumor-derived DNA was identified as a tumor-associated molecular pattern that governs inflammatory signals in the tumor microenvironment.[86] Apart from DNA recognition in the endosome (see TLR section), the innate immune system compromises a variety of cytosolic DNA receptors, comprehensively reviewed by Schlee and Hartmann.[87] In healthy eukaryotic cells, DNA is typically restricted to the nucleus and mitochondria. Its mere presence in the cytosol is indicative of non-self to the innate immune system, suggesting foreign DNA as a consequence of infection by intracellular bacteria or viruses.

Cyclic GMP-AMP synthase (cGAS) is the most widely accepted cytosolic DNA receptor.[88,89] On binding of double-stranded (ds)DNA, cGAS catalyzes the synthesis of the endogenous cyclic dinucleotide (CDN) cyclic GMP-AMP (cGAMP). As a second messenger, cGAMP activates the mitochondrial adaptor protein Stimulator of IFN Genes (STING) for potent proinflammatory downstream signaling and the release of IFN. Mice that genetically lack STING showed critically impaired priming of cytotoxic T cells and failed to reject immunogenic tumors in a preclinical transplantable model of melanoma.[86] Together with the experimental proof of tumor DNA localized in the cytosol of tumor-resident APC,[90] these data suggest that detection of tumor-derived DNA by host APC triggers inflammatory signals and IFN release that facilitate cross-priming of tumor-antigen–specific T cells. However, the molecular mechanisms how tumor DNA gains access to the cytosol of APC and whether this process involves shuttling via extracellular vesicles, such as exosomes, remains to be determined.

Detection of tumor DNA by STING seems to be detrimental not only for spontaneous but also therapy-induced antitumor T-cell responses. In preclinical models, the success of either radiation therapy or immune checkpoint blockade with anti-CTLA-4 and anti-PD1 were both dependent on the function of STING in host APC.[86,91] Targeting STING in the tumor microenvironment has thus become a prominent approach in tumor immunotherapy. However, despite promising data from preclinical mouse models, the flavonoid STING ligand 5,6-dimethylxanthenone-4-acetic acid (DMXAA) failed in a phase III clinical trial in patients with non–small cell lung cancer.[92] Follow-up studies revealed that, because of high polymorphism in the human *TMEM173* gene encoding STING, DMXAA is capable of activating murine but not human STING.[93] The development of synthetic CDN now allows for effective STING targeting in both mice and humans, with promising results in murine tumor models.[94] The CDN compounds MIW815 and MK-1454 are currently under clinical evaluation in phase I clinical trials in patients with advanced solid tumors and lymphomas (NCT03172936, NCT02675439, NCT03010176). These compounds are administered by intralesional injection, in some patients in combination with immune checkpoint blockade, targeting CTLA-4 or PD-1. Other studies have raised concerns of possible protumorigenic functions of STING. Activation of the cGAS-STING pathway can induce the immune-suppressive enzyme indolamine 2,3-dioxygenase and thus promote tumor growth.[95] These findings confirm the necessity of current strategies to combine different aspects of the immunostimulatory therapeutic network.

## RIG-I-LIKE HELICASE RECEPTOR AGONISTS

Experience with DMXAA again confirmed that the expression patterns of nucleic acid sensors differ between species, which frequently skews the translation of preclinical results into human disease. The antiviral RIG-I–like helicases (RLH) family of cytosolic RNA receptors is broadly expressed in both murine and human immune as well as nonimmune cells. On ligand binding, RLH can induce proinflammatory cyto-kines, ASC-dependent inflammasome activation,[96–98] and IFN release[99,100] via the mitochondrial adapter molecule MAVS (mitochondrial antiviral-signaling protein; also IPS1 or VISA). Its eponymous member retinoic acid-inducible gene I (RIG-I) pri-marily detects short cytosolic dsRNA with a free 5′-triphosphate group (pppRNA).[100] RNA is generated by enzymatic 3′ to 5′ linkage of triphosphate nucleotides, which inevitably leaves a free triphosphate group at the 5′ end. Endogenous RNA is synthe-sized in the nucleus and before translocation to the cytosol is further processed (eg, by 5′ capping) to hide the 5′-triphosphate ends from the host's immune system. Uncapped RNA with an accessible 5′-triphosphate in the cytosol indicates non-self RNA that has formed outside the nucleus and, thus, is an alarm signal to the host indicating viral replication or intracellular bacteria. Activation of the RNA recep-tor melanoma differentiation-associated protein 5 is less well characterized but seems to involve the detection of long dsRNA with complex secondary structures. How the immune system discriminates self from non-self nucleic acids has been extensively reviewed elsewhere.[87]

Using virus infection models, it has been shown that detection of viral RNA and sub-sequent RIG-I signaling can potently induce the cross-priming of cytotoxic T cells.[101] Harnessing antiviral mechanisms in preclinical cancer models by selective activation of the RIG-I pathway with pppRNA has been shown to result in growth inhibition of pre-established tumors, involving dendritic cell–mediated IFN production and other innate effector mechanisms such as activation of NK cells.[102] Because detection of pppRNAs is largely independent of their nucleotide sequence, bifunctional pppRNA molecules have been designed to additionally facilitate gene silencing via RNA inter-ference. Such small interfering (si)RNAs harboring a 5′-triphosphate group that target oncogenes such as anti-apoptotic B-cell lymphoma 2 or transforming growth factor β have proven high antitumor activity in different murine cancer models.[102,103]

RIG-I is commonly expressed not only in host immune cells but also in tumor cells.[102] Tumor-intrinsic RIG-I activation by specific pppRNA compounds has been found to trigger a strong and cell-autonomous induction of programmed tumor cell death that involves cleavage of the executioner caspase-3.[102,104] This pathway was found to be particularly active in malignant cells and resulted in an immunogenic form of tumor cell death, which was associated with potent cross-priming of tumor-specific cytotoxic T cells in vitro.[14] Thanks to these various antitumor functions, target-ing RLH in the tumor microenvironment has evolved as a promising immunothera-peutic approach. Intralesional application of the synthetic RIG-I ligand RGT100-PEI in patients with advanced solid tumors and lymphomas is currently being evaluated in a phase I/II clinical trial (NCT03065023).

Under certain conditions, endogenous RIG-I ligands seem to also contribute to the development of antitumor immune responses. Induction of tumor cell apoptosis following genotoxic therapy such as radiation or chemotherapeutic agents has been suggested to be dependent on the translocation of small non-coding RNAs into the cytosol, where they activate RIG-I signaling and IFN release in tumor cells.[105] The in-hibitor of DNA methyltransferases 5-azacytidine is approved for the treatment of mye-lodysplastic syndrome and acute myeloid leukemias. Two independent studies have recently shown that 5-azacytidine treatment of tumor cells can result in the enhanced transcription of endogenous retroviral elements (ERVs) that are stably integrated in the tumor cell genome.[105,106] Detection of ERV mRNA by RLHs induced an antiviral IFN response that synergized with immune checkpoint blockade. Whether detection of endogenous RLH ligands contribute to the effectiveness of other cancer treatments will have to be clarified by future studies.

Furthermore, oncolytic virus therapy may involve signaling via nucleic acid receptors. Several preclinical studies suggest that therapeutic efficacy of oncolytic viruses is not only due to direct infection-mediated tumor cell lysis, but also critically depends on subsequent activation of innate and adaptive antitumor immunity.[107] Talimogene laherparepvec (T-VEC) is a genetically engineered, oncogenic herpes simplex virus 1 (HSV-1) that encodes for human granulocyte macrophage colony-stimulating factor and is approved for intralesional treatment in patients with advanced melanoma. HSV-1 replication intermediates can be detected via RLH[108]; however, whether detection of oncolytic virus RNA by RLH or other nucleic acid sensors contributes to its systemic antitumor efficacy remains to be determined.

## ANTIBODIES FOR INNATE STIMULATION

The myeloid cell compartment of the innate immune system is intrinsically intertwined with the induction of adaptive immunity. Thus, strategies targeting these cells will influence the development of specific immunity. Such approaches include modulation of suppressive cells, for example, myeloid-derived suppressor cells or tumor-associated macrophages as well as the direct use of dendritic cell vaccines loaded with tumor antigens.[109–111]

By contrast, innate immune effector cells, such as NK cells, can recognize and lyse cancer cells without prior licensing by APCs, as required for cells of the adaptive immune system.[112,113] Activation of NK cells toward a given target cell can principally come in 2 flavors: engagement of activating receptors, for example, CD16 or NKG2D, or the detection of alterations in receptor or ligand expression.[113] An example for the latter is the loss of MHC-I on cancer cells, which is a mechanism known to inhibit NK-cell function via KIRs. The latter is a highly specialized and diverse system because different receptors will sense different HLA types. According to this notion, adequate manipulation of NK-cell function can result in effective antitumor activity.[113]

As such, elotuzumab, an immunostimulatory monoclonal antibody targeting signaling lymphocytic activation molecule F7 (SLAMF7), has been approved for the treatment of refractory multiple myeloma.[114] SLAMF7 is expressed on both NK and myeloma cells. Elotuzumab exerts its function via dual mechanisms by (1) directly activating NK cells and (2) mediating antibody-dependent cellular cytotoxicity (ADCC) through CD16.[115] Fc-competent monoclonal antibodies, in general, may nonspecifically recruit FcγR-positive cells such as NK cells and exert ADCC-dependent antitumor activity. Examples would include the CD20 antibodies rituximab or obinutuzumab for the treatment of different B-cell lymphomas and acute B-lymphocytic leukemias.[116,117] Because the clinical contribution of such accessory cells to the activity of these antibodies is controversial, we refer the interested reader to recent reviews on the topic.[118,119]

Another strategy is the direct therapeutic use of NK cells. Autologous NK cells can be harvested by leukapheresis, then expanded and genetically manipulated for enhanced specificity and function, before reinfusion into the patient.[120] Based on compelling preclinical evidence, clinical trials currently evaluate activated NK cells, NK cells genetically modified with chimeric antigen receptors, or off-the-shelf NK cells, in different antineoplastic indications (reviewed in[120]).

In analogy to success in reinvigorating and activating adaptive immune responses by targeting the immune checkpoints CTLA-4 and PD-1,[121] several trials are under way to evaluate agents (re-)activating NK cells for cancer treatment. NK cells can be boosted using recombinant IL-15, which can enhance NK-cell activation and cytotoxicity against cancer cells.[122] As a caveat, IL-15 also targets other IL-15 receptor-expressing cell populations such as T cells; thus, the effects that might be seen in ongoing clinical trials will be difficult to ascribe to NK cells only.[123] Different forms of recombinant IL-15 with variations in their biophysical properties are currently under development.[113] The strategy of NK-cell re-engagement by blocking NK-suppressive molecules, using monoclonal antibodies against KIR, NKG2A, TIM-3, and TIGIT, is currently under investigation in several early clinical trials.[113] Finally, specific retargeting of NK cells with bispecific antibodies, binding CD16 on the NK-cell side and a tumor-associated antigen on the other side, have been developed and have entered clinical trials (NCT03214666, NCT03192202).[21] These ongoing investigations will reveal whether and how NK cells can be successfully used for cancer treatment.

## OUTLOOK AND SUMMARY

Unlike the adaptive immune system, which—with the advent of T cell–targeting cancer therapies—has entered clinical practice, the use of strategies harnessing different components of the innate immune system is still in its infancy. With the exception of the TLR7/8 agonist imiquimod, no compound specifically targeting a component of the innate immune system has yet reached approval as a single agent in cancer treatment. In the present review, we provide a broad overview of current and past developments in this growing field. An important consideration to bear in mind is that most, if not all, of the outlined strategies will ultimately influence the induction of specific immunity if successful. Designing strategies targeting either arm of the immune system will most likely impact on the other arm. Dichotomy in terms of mode of action can only be safely discriminated in mouse models allowing depletion of each compartment at a time.

The success of immune oncology has boosted the development of additional strategies, also including combination therapies.[124] The research area of innate immunity has benefited from this development in both single-agent and combination treatment after a series of earlier negative results from clinical trials. Ongoing investigation will show whether some of the aforementioned experimental strategies might find a place in clinical oncology.

## ACKNOWLEDGMENTS

This study was supported by grants from the Bundesministerium für Bildung und Forschung VIP + grant ONKATTRACT (to S. Kobold), the Dres. Carl Maximilian and Carl Manfred Bayer-Foundation (to S. Heidegger), the Else Kröner-Fresenius-Stiftung (to S. Kobold and S. Heidegger), the Ernst-Jung-Stiftung (to S. Kobold), the European Research Council Starting Grant (grant number 756017 to S. Kobold), the German Cancer Aid (to S. Kobold and S. Heidegger), the German Research Foundation (DFG) (DU1522/1-1 and SFB1123 to P. Düwell), the international doctoral program "i-Target: Immunotargeting of cancer" funded by the Elite Network of Bavaria (to S. Kobold), the LMU Munich's Institutional Strategy LMUexcellent within the framework of the German Excellence Initiative (to S. Kobold), the Marie-Sklodowska-Curie "Training Network for the Immunotherapy of Cancer (IMMUTRAIN)" funded by the H2020 program of the European Union (to S. Kobold), and the Melanoma Research Alliance (grant number 409510 to S. Kobold).

## REFERENCES

1. Sharma P, Allison JP. The future of immune checkpoint therapy. Science 2015; 348(6230):56–61.

2. Teng MW, Ngiow SF, Ribas A, et al. Classifying cancers based on T-cell infiltration and PD-L1. Cancer Res 2015;75(11):2139–45.
3. Sharma P, Wagner K, Wolchok JD, et al. Novel cancer immunotherapy agents with survival benefit: recent successes and next steps. Nat Rev Cancer 2011; 11(11):805–12.
4. Freeman GJ, Long AJ, Iwai Y, et al. Engagement of the PD-1 immunoinhibitory receptor by a novel B7 family member leads to negative regulation of lymphocyte activation. J Exp Med 2000;192(7):1027–34.
5. Dong H, Strome SE, Salomao DR, et al. Tumor-associated B7-H1 promotes T-cell apoptosis: a potential mechanism of immune evasion. Nat Med 2002;8(8): 793–800.
6. Dudley ME, Wunderlich JR, Robbins PF, et al. Cancer regression and autoimmunity in patients after clonal repopulation with antitumor lymphocytes. Science 2002;298(5594):850–4.
7. Rosenberg SA, Yang JC, Sherry RM, et al. Durable complete responses in heavily pretreated patients with metastatic melanoma using T-cell transfer immunotherapy. Clin Cancer Res 2011;17(13):4550–7.
8. Yang JC, Rosenberg SA. Current approaches to the adoptive immunotherapy of cancer. Adv Exp Med Biol 1988;233:459–67.
9. Morgan RA, Dudley ME, Wunderlich JR, et al. Cancer regression in patients after transfer of genetically engineered lymphocytes. Science 2006;314(5796): 126–9.
10. Kalos M, Levine BL, Porter DL, et al. T cells with chimeric antigen receptors have potent antitumor effects and can establish memory in patients with advanced leukemia. Sci Transl Med 2011;3(95):95ra73.
11. Yan Y, Kumar AB, Finnes H, et al. Combining immune checkpoint inhibitors with conventional cancer therapy. Front Immunol 2018;9:1739.
12. Zitvogel L, Kepp O, Kroemer G. Decoding cell death signals in inflammation and immunity. Cell 2010;140(6):798–804.
13. Tang D, Kang R, Coyne CB, et al. PAMPs and DAMPs: signal 0s that spur autophagy and immunity. Immunol Rev 2012;249(1):158–75.
14. Duewell P, Steger A, Lohr H, et al. RIG-I-like helicases induce immunogenic cell death of pancreatic cancer cells and sensitize tumors toward killing by CD8(+) T cells. Cell Death Differ 2014;21(12):1825–37.
15. Ivarsson MA, Michaelsson J, Fauriat C. Activating killer cell Ig-like receptors in health and disease. Front Immunol 2014;5:184.
16. Lowry LE, Zehring WA. Potentiation of natural killer cells for cancer immunotherapy: a review of literature. Front Immunol 2017;8:1061.
17. Mellman I, Coukos G, Dranoff G. Cancer immunotherapy comes of age. Nature 2011;480(7378):480–9.
18. O'Neill LA, Golenbock D, Bowie AG. The history of Toll-like receptors - redefining innate immunity. Nat Rev Immunol 2013;13(6):453–60.
19. Roach JC, Glusman G, Rowen L, et al. The evolution of vertebrate Toll-like receptors. Proc Natl Acad Sci U S A 2005;102(27):9577–82.
20. Uematsu S, Akira S. Toll-like receptors and innate immunity. J Mol Med 2006; 84(9):712–25.
21. Engelhardt R, Mackensen A, Galanos C. Phase I trial of intravenously administered endotoxin (Salmonella abortus equi) in cancer patients. Cancer Res 1991; 51(10):2524–30.
22. Wiemann B, Starnes CO. Coley's toxins, tumor necrosis factor and cancer research: a historical perspective. Pharmacol Ther 1994;64(3):529–64.

23. Vacchelli E, Galluzzi L, Eggermont A, et al. Trial watch: FDA-approved Toll-like receptor agonists for cancer therapy. Oncoimmunology 2012;1(6):894–907.

24. Kobold S, Wiedemann G, Rothenfusser S, et al. Modes of action of TLR7 agonists in cancer therapy. Immunotherapy 2014;6(10):1085–95.

25. Manegold C, van Zandwijk N, Szczesna A, et al. A phase III randomized study of gemcitabine and cisplatin with or without PF-3512676 (TLR9 agonist) as first-line treatment of advanced non-small-cell lung cancer. Ann Oncol 2012;23(1):72–7.

26. Gross CJ, Mishra R, Schneider KS, et al. K(+) efflux-independent NLRP3 inflammasome activation by small molecules targeting mitochondria. Immunity 2016;45(4):761–73.

27. Salazar LG, Lu H, Reichow JL, et al. Topical imiquimod plus nab-paclitaxel for breast cancer cutaneous metastases: a phase 2 clinical trial. JAMA Oncol 2017;3(7):969–73.

28. Aranda F, Vacchelli E, Obrist F, et al. Trial watch: toll-like receptor agonists in oncological indications. Oncoimmunology 2014;3:e29179.

29. Vacchelli E, Eggermont A, Sautes-Fridman C, et al. Trial watch: toll-like receptor agonists for cancer therapy. Oncoimmunology 2013;2(8):e25238.

30. Iribarren K, Bloy N, Buque A, et al. Trial watch: immunostimulation with toll-like receptor agonists in cancer therapy. Oncoimmunology 2016;5(3):e1088631.

31. Skinner SR, Szarewski A, Romanowski B, et al. Efficacy, safety, and immunogenicity of the human papillomavirus 16/18 AS04-adjuvanted vaccine in women older than 25 years: 4-year interim follow-up of the phase 3, double-blind, randomised controlled VIVIANE study. Lancet 2014;384(9961):2213–27.

32. Sahin U, Derhovanessian E, Miller M, et al. Personalized RNA mutanome vaccines mobilize poly-specific therapeutic immunity against cancer. Nature 2017;547(7662):222–6.

33. Parlato M, Yeretssian G. NOD-like receptors in intestinal homeostasis and epithelial tissue repair. Int J Mol Sci 2014;15(6):9594–627.

34. Weinheimer-Haus EM, Mirza RE, Koh TJ. Nod-like receptor protein-3 inflammasome plays an important role during early stages of wound healing. PLoS One 2015;10(3):e0119106.

35. Ting JP, Lovering RC, Alnemri ES, et al. The NLR gene family: a standard nomenclature. Immunity 2008;28(3):285–7.

36. Chamaillard M, Hashimoto M, Horie Y, et al. An essential role for NOD1 in host recognition of bacterial peptidoglycan containing diaminopimelic acid. Nat Immunol 2003;4(7):702–7.

37. Girardin SE, Boneca IG, Viala J, et al. Nod2 is a general sensor of peptidoglycan through muramyl dipeptide (MDP) detection. J Biol Chem 2003;278(11):8869–72.

38. Ogura Y, Lala S, Xin W, et al. Expression of NOD2 in Paneth cells: a possible link to Crohn's ileitis. Gut 2003;52(11):1591–7.

39. Chen GY, Shaw MH, Redondo G, et al. The innate immune receptor Nod1 protects the intestine from inflammation-induced tumorigenesis. Cancer Res 2008;68(24):10060–7.

40. Couturier-Maillard A, Secher T, Rehman A, et al. NOD2-mediated dysbiosis predisposes mice to transmissible colitis and colorectal cancer. J Clin Invest 2013;123(2):700–11.

41. Wang P, Zhang L, Jiang JM, et al. Association of NOD1 and NOD2 genes polymorphisms with Helicobacter pylori related gastric cancer in a Chinese population. World J Gastroenterol 2012;18(17):2112–20.

42. da Silva Correia J, Miranda Y, Austin-Brown N, et al. Nod1-dependent control of tumor growth. Proc Natl Acad Sci U S A 2006;103(6):1840–5.

43. Kutikhin AG. Role of NOD1/CARD4 and NOD2/CARD15 gene polymorphisms in cancer etiology. Hum Immunol 2011;72(10):955–68.

44. Martinon F, Burns K, Tschopp J. The inflammasome: a molecular platform triggering activation of inflammatory caspases and processing of proIL-beta. Mol Cell 2002;10(2):417–26.

45. Latz E, Xiao TS, Stutz A. Activation and regulation of the inflammasomes. Nat Rev Immunol 2013;13(6):397–411.

46. Miao EA, Rajan JV, Aderem A. Caspase-1-induced pyroptotic cell death. Immunol Rev 2011;243(1):206–14.

47. Allen IC, TeKippe EM, Woodford RM, et al. The NLRP3 inflammasome functions as a negative regulator of tumorigenesis during colitis-associated cancer. J Exp Med 2010;207(5):1045–56.

48. Normand S, Delanoye-Crespin A, Bressenot A, et al. Nod-like receptor pyrin domain-containing protein 6 (NLRP6) controls epithelial self-renewal and colorectal carcinogenesis upon injury. Proc Natl Acad Sci U S A 2011;108(23): 9601–6.

49. Huhn S, da Silva Filho MI, Sanmuganantham T, et al. Coding variants in NOD-like receptors: an association study on risk and survival of colorectal cancer. PLoS One 2018;13(6):e0199350.

50. Steidl C, Shah SP, Woolcock BW, et al. MHC class II transactivator CIITA is a recurrent gene fusion partner in lymphoid cancers. Nature 2011;471(7338): 377–81.

51. Chen GY, Liu M, Wang F, et al. A functional role for Nlrp6 in intestinal inflammation and tumorigenesis. J Immunol 2011;186(12):7187–94.

52. Ohno S, Kinoshita T, Ohno Y, et al. Expression of NLRP7 (PYPAF3, NALP7) protein in endometrial cancer tissues. Anticancer Res 2008;28(4C):2493–7.

53. Okada K, Hirota E, Mizutani Y, et al. Oncogenic role of NALP7 in testicular seminomas. Cancer Sci 2004;95(12):949–54.

54. Vance RE. The NAIP/NLRC4 inflammasomes. Curr Opin Immunol 2015;32:84–9.

55. Martinon F, Petrilli V, Mayor A, et al. Gout-associated uric acid crystals activate the NALP3 inflammasome. Nature 2006;440(7081):237–41.

56. Heneka MT, Kummer MP, Stutz A, et al. NLRP3 is activated in Alzheimer's disease and contributes to pathology in APP/PS1 mice. Nature 2013;493(7434): 674–8.

57. Duewell P, Kono H, Rayner KJ, et al. NLRP3 inflammasomes are required for atherogenesis and activated by cholesterol crystals. Nature 2010;464(7293): 1357–61.

58. Shimada K, Crother TR, Karlin J, et al. Oxidized mitochondrial DNA activates the NLRP3 inflammasome during apoptosis. Immunity 2012;36(3):401–14.

59. Zhou R, Tardivel A, Thorens B, et al. Thioredoxin-interacting protein links oxidative stress to inflammasome activation. Nat Immunol 2010;11(2):136–40.

60. Petrilli V, Papin S, Dostert C, et al. Activation of the NALP3 inflammasome is triggered by low intracellular potassium concentration. Cell Death Differ 2007;14(9): 1583–9.

61. Mariathasan S, Weiss DS, Newton K, et al. Cryopyrin activates the inflammasome in response to toxins and ATP. Nature 2006;440(7081):228–32.

62. Dunn JH, Ellis LZ, Fujita M. Inflammasomes as molecular mediators of inflammation and cancer: potential role in melanoma. Cancer Lett 2012;314(1):24–33.

63. Tu S, Bhagat G, Cui G, et al. Overexpression of interleukin-1beta induces gastric inflammation and cancer and mobilizes myeloid-derived suppressor cells in mice. Cancer Cell 2008;14(5):408–19.

64. Chow MT, Tschopp J, Moller A, et al. NLRP3 promotes inflammation-induced skin cancer but is dispensable for asbestos-induced mesothelioma. Immunol Cell Biol 2012;90(10):983–6.

65. Zaki MH, Vogel P, Body-Malapel M, et al. IL-18 production downstream of the Nlrp3 inflammasome confers protection against colorectal tumor formation. J Immunol 2010;185(8):4912–20.

66. Tarhini AA, Millward M, Mainwaring P, et al. A phase 2, randomized study of SB-485232, rhIL-18, in patients with previously untreated metastatic melanoma. Cancer 2009;115(4):859–68.

67. Ridker PM, Everett BM, Thuren T, et al. Antiinflammatory therapy with canakinumab for atherosclerotic disease. N Engl J Med 2017;377(12):1119–31.

68. Ridker PM, MacFadyen JG, Thuren T, et al. Effect of interleukin-1beta inhibition with canakinumab on incident lung cancer in patients with atherosclerosis: exploratory results from a randomised, double-blind, placebo-controlled trial. Lancet 2017;390(10105):1833–42.

69. Pelegrin P, Surprenant A. Pannexin-1 mediates large pore formation and interleukin-1beta release by the ATP-gated P2X7 receptor. EMBO J 2006; 25(21):5071–82.

70. Gombault A, Baron L, Couillin I. ATP release and purinergic signaling in NLRP3 inflammasome activation. Front Immunol 2012;3:414.

71. Li H, Willingham SB, Ting JP, et al. Cutting edge: inflammasome activation by alum and alum's adjuvant effect are mediated by NLRP3. J Immunol 2008; 181(1):17–21.

72. Marty-Roix R, Vladimer GI, Pouliot K, et al. Identification of QS-21 as an Inflammasome-activating molecular component of saponin adjuvants. J Biol Chem 2016;291(3):1123–36.

73. Franchi L, Nunez G. The Nlrp3 inflammasome is critical for aluminium hydroxide-mediated IL-1beta secretion but dispensable for adjuvant activity. Eur J Immunol 2008;38(8):2085–9.

74. Morein B. Iscom–an immunostimulating complex. Arzneimittelforschung 1987; 37(12):1418.

75. Jacobs C, Duewell P, Heckelsmiller K, et al. An ISCOM vaccine combined with a TLR9 agonist breaks immune evasion mediated by regulatory T cells in an orthotopic model of pancreatic carcinoma. Int J Cancer 2011;128(4):897–907.

76. Maraskovsky E, Schnurr M, Wilson NS, et al. Development of prophylactic and therapeutic vaccines using the ISCOMATRIX adjuvant. Immunol Cell Biol 2009; 87(5):371–6.

77. Wilson NS, Duewell P, Yang B, et al. Inflammasome-dependent and -independent IL-18 production mediates immunity to the ISCOMATRIX adjuvant. J Immunol 2014;192(7):3259–68.

78. Duewell P, Kisser U, Heckelsmiller K, et al. ISCOMATRIX adjuvant combines immune activation with antigen delivery to dendritic cells in vivo leading to effective cross-priming of CD8+ T cells. J Immunol 2011;187(1):55–63.

79. Maraskovsky E, Sjolander S, Drane DP, et al. NY-ESO-1 protein formulated in ISCOMATRIX adjuvant is a potent anticancer vaccine inducing both humoral and CD8+ t-cell-mediated immunity and protection against NY-ESO-1+ tumors. Clin Cancer Res 2004;10(8):2879–90.

80. Robson NC, McAlpine T, Knights AJ, et al. Processing and cross-presentation of individual HLA-A, -B, or -C epitopes from NY-ESO-1 or an HLA-A epitope for Melan-A differ according to the mode of antigen delivery. Blood 2010;116(2): 218–25.
81. McKenzie A, Watt M, Gittleson C. ISCOMATRIX() vaccines: safety in human clinical studies. Hum Vaccin 2010;6(3) [pii:10754].
82. Coll RC, Robertson AA, Chae JJ, et al. A small-molecule inhibitor of the NLRP3 inflammasome for the treatment of inflammatory diseases. Nat Med 2015;21(3): 248–55.
83. Chen L, Huang CF, Li YC, et al. Blockage of the NLRP3 inflammasome by MCC950 improves anti-tumor immune responses in head and neck squamous cell carcinoma. Cell Mol Life Sci 2018;75(11):2045–58.
84. Mullard A. Can innate immune system targets turn up the heat on 'cold' tumours? Nat Rev Drug Discov 2018;17(1):3–5.
85. Chen GY, Nunez G. Sterile inflammation: sensing and reacting to damage. Nat Rev Immunol 2010;10(12):826–37.
86. Woo SR, Fuertes MB, Corrales L, et al. STING-dependent cytosolic DNA sensing mediates innate immune recognition of immunogenic tumors. Immunity 2014;41(5):830–42.
87. Schlee M, Hartmann G. Discriminating self from non-self in nucleic acid sensing. Nat Rev Immunol 2016;16(9):566–80.
88. Sun L, Wu J, Du F, et al. Cyclic GMP-AMP synthase is a cytosolic DNA sensor that activates the type I interferon pathway. Science 2013;339(6121):786–91.
89. Wu J, Sun L, Chen X, et al. Cyclic GMP-AMP is an endogenous second messenger in innate immune signaling by cytosolic DNA. Science 2013; 339(6121):826–30.
90. Klarquist J, Hennies CM, Lehn MA, et al. STING-mediated DNA sensing promotes antitumor and autoimmune responses to dying cells. J Immunol 2014; 193(12):6124–34.
91. Deng L, Liang H, Xu M, et al. STING-dependent cytosolic DNA sensing promotes radiation-induced type i interferon-dependent antitumor immunity in immunogenic tumors. Immunity 2014;41(5):843–52.
92. Lara PN Jr, Douillard JY, Nakagawa K, et al. Randomized phase III placebo-controlled trial of carboplatin and paclitaxel with or without the vascular disrupting agent vadimezan (ASA404) in advanced non-small-cell lung cancer. J Clin Oncol 2011;29(22):2965–71.
93. Conlon J, Burdette DL, Sharma S, et al. Mouse, but not human STING, binds and signals in response to the vascular disrupting agent 5,6-dimethylxanthenone-4-acetic acid. J Immunol 2013;190(10):5216–25.
94. Corrales L, Glickman LH, McWhirter SM, et al. Direct activation of STING in the tumor microenvironment leads to potent and systemic tumor regression and immunity. Cell Rep 2015;11(7):1018–30.
95. Huang L, Li L, Lemos H, et al. Cutting edge: DNA sensing via the STING adaptor in myeloid dendritic cells induces potent tolerogenic responses. J Immunol 2013;191(7):3509–13.
96. Poeck H, Bscheider M, Gross O, et al. Recognition of RNA virus by RIG-I results in activation of CARD9 and inflammasome signaling for interleukin 1 beta production. Nat Immunol 2010;11(1):63–9.
97. Franchi L, Eigenbrod T, Munoz-Planillo R, et al. Cytosolic double-stranded RNA activates the NLRP3 inflammasome via MAVS-induced membrane permeabilization and K+ efflux. J Immunol 2014;193(8):4214–22.

98. Pothlichet J, Meunier I, Davis BK, et al. Type I IFN triggers RIG-I/TLR3/NLRP3-dependent inflammasome activation in influenza A virus infected cells. PLoS Pathog 2013;9(4):e1003256.

99. Goubau D, Schlee M, Deddouche S, et al. Antiviral immunity via RIG-I-mediated recognition of RNA bearing 5'-diphosphates. Nature 2014;514(7522):372–5.

100. Hornung V, Ellegast J, Kim S, et al. 5'-Triphosphate RNA is the ligand for RIG-I. Science 2006;314(5801):994–7.

101. Hochheiser K, Klein M, Gottschalk C, et al. Cutting edge: the RIG-I ligand 3pRNA potently improves CTL cross-priming and facilitates antiviral vaccination. J Immunol 2016;196(6):2439–43.

102. Poeck H, Besch R, Maihoefer C, et al. 5'-Triphosphate-siRNA: turning gene silencing and Rig-I activation against melanoma. Nat Med 2008;14(11):1256–63.

103. Ellermeier J, Wei J, Duewell P, et al. Therapeutic efficacy of bifunctional siRNA combining TGF-beta1 silencing with RIG-I activation in pancreatic cancer. Cancer Res 2013;73(6):1709–20.

104. Besch R, Poeck H, Hohenauer T, et al. Proapoptotic signaling induced by RIG-I and MDA-5 results in type I interferon-independent apoptosis in human melanoma cells. J Clin Invest 2009;119(8):2399–411.

105. Ranoa DR, Parekh AD, Pitroda SP, et al. Cancer therapies activate RIG-I-like receptor pathway through endogenous non-coding RNAs. Oncotarget 2016;7(18):26496–515.

106. Roulois D, Loo Yau H, Singhania R, et al. DNA-demethylating agents target colorectal cancer cells by inducing viral mimicry by endogenous transcripts. Cell 2015;162(5):961–73.

107. Turnbull S, West EJ, Scott KJ, et al. Evidence for oncolytic virotherapy: where have we got to and where are we going? Viruses 2015;7(12):6291–312.

108. Melchjorsen J, Rintahaka J, Soby S, et al. Early innate recognition of herpes simplex virus in human primary macrophages is mediated via the MDA5/MAVS-dependent and MDA5/MAVS/RNA polymerase III-independent pathways. J Virol 2010;84(21):11350–8.

109. Cotechini T, Medler TR, Coussens LM. Myeloid cells as targets for therapy in solid tumors. Cancer J 2015;21(4):343–50.

110. Fleming V, Hu X, Weber R, et al. Targeting myeloid-derived suppressor cells to bypass tumor-induced immunosuppression. Front Immunol 2018;9:398.

111. Kantoff PW, Higano CS, Shore ND, et al. Sipuleucel-T immunotherapy for castration-resistant prostate cancer. N Engl J Med 2010;363(5):411–22.

112. Bachanova V, Miller JS. NK cells in therapy of cancer. Crit Rev Oncog 2014;19(1–2):133–41.

113. Cooley S, Parham P, Miller JS. Strategies to activate NK cells to prevent relapse and induce remission following hematopoietic stem cell transplantation. Blood 2018;131(10):1053–62.

114. Lonial S, Dimopoulos M, Palumbo A, et al. Elotuzumab therapy for relapsed or refractory multiple myeloma. N Engl J Med 2015;373(7):621–31.

115. Collins SM, Bakan CE, Swartzel GD, et al. Elotuzumab directly enhances NK cell cytotoxicity against myeloma via CS1 ligation: evidence for augmented NK cell function complementing ADCC. Cancer Immunol Immunother 2013;62(12):1841–9.

116. Kobold S, Lutkens T, Cao Y, et al. Autoantibodies against tumor-related antigens: incidence and biologic significance. Hum Immunol 2010;71(7):643–51.

117. Meyer S, Evers M, Jansen JHM, et al. New insights in Type I and II CD20 antibody mechanisms-of-action with a panel of novel CD20 antibodies. Br J Haematol 2018;180(6):808–20.
118. Redman JM, Hill EM, AlDeghaither D, et al. Mechanisms of action of therapeutic antibodies for cancer. Mol Immunol 2015;67(2 Pt A):28–45.
119. Rajasekaran N, Chester C, Yonezawa A, et al. Enhancement of antibody-dependent cell mediated cytotoxicity: a new era in cancer treatment. Immunotargets Ther 2015;4:91–100.
120. Daher M, Rezvani K. Next generation natural killer cells for cancer immunotherapy: the promise of genetic engineering. Curr Opin Immunol 2018;51: 146–53.
121. Kobold S, Krackhardt A, Schlosser H, et al. Immuno-oncology: a brief overview. Dtsch Med Wochenschr 2018;143(14):1006–13 [in German].
122. Margolin K, Morishima C, Velcheti V, et al. Phase I trial of ALT-803, a novel recombinant interleukin-15 complex, in patients with advanced solid tumors. Clin Cancer Res 2018;24(22):5552–61.
123. Conlon KC, Lugli E, Welles HC, et al. Redistribution, hyperproliferation, activation of natural killer cells and CD8 T cells, and cytokine production during first-in-human clinical trial of recombinant human interleukin-15 in patients with cancer. J Clin Oncol 2015;33(1):74–82.
124. Tang J, Shalabi A, Hubbard-Lucey VM. Comprehensive analysis of the clinical immuno-oncology landscape. Ann Oncol 2018;29(1):84–91.
125. Molfetta R, Quatrini L, Santoni A, et al. Regulation of NKG2D-dependent NK cell functions: the Yin and the Yang of receptor endocytosis. Int J Mol Sci 2017;18(8) [pii:E1677].

# Radiation Therapy and Immune Modulation

Jonathan E. Leeman, MD, Jonathan D. Schoenfeld, MD, MPhil, MPH*

## KEYWORDS

- Radiotherapy • Immune checkpoint blockade • Immunotherapy • Abscopal effect

## KEY POINTS

- Radiotherapy has known immunomodulatory effects and there is a strong preclinical rationale for combining radiotherapy with immunotherapies to enhance both locoregional and systemic effects.
- Recent prospective trials evaluating radiotherapy/immunotherapy combinations are reporting encouraging data on safety and efficacy in the definitive setting for many cancer types.
- Randomized studies assessing systemic effects in the metastatic setting with the addition of radiotherapy to immunotherapies are ongoing and have demonstrated promising early data.

## PRECLINICAL RATIONALE FOR COMBINING RADIOTHERAPY WITH CHECKPOINT BLOCKADE

In addition to the 4 Rs of radiobiology (repair, reassortment, repopulation, and reoxygenation), which are thought to underlie the cellular mechanisms in response to radiotherapy, immune effects are also responsible, at least in part, for tumor control following radiotherapy. Clinically, it has been observed that immunocompromised patients may experience inferior tumor control after radiotherapy.[1] In a mouse fibrosarcoma model, immunosuppression with whole-body irradiation or thymectomy led to a significantly higher subsequent radiation dose needed for tumor control.[2] Similarly, in a syngeneic mouse model of head and neck squamous cell carcinoma (HNSCC), tumors were only cleared with radiotherapy and cisplatin in immune-competent mice, whereas immune suppression blunted the efficacy of radiotherapy.[3] More specifically, reduction of tumor burden following radiation therapy (RT) to ablative doses has been found to depend on T cell responses.[4] Irradiated cells are more capable of presenting

Disclosure Statement: J.D. Schoenfeld acknowledges research funding from BMS, Merck, and consulting fees from BMS, Debiopharm Group, AZ, Nanobiotix, and Tilos Therapeutics.
Department of Radiation Oncology, Dana Farber Cancer Institute, Brigham and Women's Hospital, 450 Brookline Avenue, Boston, MA 02215, USA
* Corresponding author.
E-mail address: jonathan_schoenfeld@dfci.harvard.edu

tumor antigens, leading to development of T cell responses and secretion of interferon-gamma (IFN-$\gamma$) in draining lymph nodes.[5] Irradiated tumors also demonstrate higher numbers of tumor-infiltrating lymphocytes and immune activation within tumor-draining lymph nodes.[5] Response to chemotherapy and radiation has been shown to rely on activation of antigen-specific T cell immunity through Toll-like receptor 4 signaling in dendritic cells.[6] In fact, the dendritic cell type 1 IFN pathway likely plays a central role in the efficacy of radiotherapy. Radiation enhances the cross-priming ability of tumor-infiltrating dendritic cells in wild-type mice but not type I IFN receptor-deficient mice.[7] Radiotherapy also may expose tumor antigens or neoantigens, induce cell surface expression of major histocompatibility complex class I (MHC class I) molecules, and improve cytotoxic T lymphocyte recognition of MHC class I molecules,[8] in this way, acting as an in situ vaccine. The type 1 IFN response in this context seems to be mediated in part by the cGAS-STING intracellular DNA-sensing pathway.[9,10] Taken together, this body of evidence indicates that tumor cell death and eradication following radiotherapy is in large part mediated by both innate and adaptive immune responses. These effects may therefore result in immune recognition of irradiated tumors and associated antigens that may potentially be enhanced with immunotherapies, such as immune checkpoint blockade (ICB).

Multiple preclinical studies have elucidated synergistic effects with administration of radiotherapy and various immunotherapies including ICB with anti-CTLA4[11,12] and anti-PD1/PDL1 agents.[13-16] Twyman-Saint Victor and colleagues[17] explored immunologic mechanisms underlying radiotherapy in combination with dual anti-CTLA4 and anti-PD1/PDL1 blockade, and found that anti-CTLA4 blockade primarily inhibited regulatory T cells (Treg) resulting in an increased CD8/Treg ratio, whereas radiation enhanced the diversity of the T cell repertoire in tumor-associated lymphocytes; whereas, anti-PDL1 blockade reversed T cell exhaustion and promoted an elevated CD8/Treg ratio. The combination of radiotherapy, and anti-CTLA4 and anti-PD1/PDL1 blockade, resulted in superior outcomes compared with radiotherapy with either agent alone. These reports have collectively demonstrated enhanced local effects of radiotherapy with ICB, but also systemic effects with destruction of non-irradiated distant lesions and improved survival in mice. However, for multiple reasons, including the inherent immunologic differences between species and wide discrepancies in tumor sizes between mice and humans, the findings from murine models cannot be extrapolated to human cancers without clinical validation.

## ABSCOPAL EFFECTS

The promise of synergy between radiotherapy and ICB lies partially in the observation of "abscopal" effects whereby disease outside of the radiation field is affected by local irradiation, which is thought to be mediated by systemic immunomodulation. Multiple case series have reported regression of systemic disease with RT and immunotherapy combinations or the initiation of radiotherapy during ICB, most frequently in patients with melanoma.[18-22]

In an effort to identify more formal evidence for abscopal effects, 2 studies were presented at the American Society of Clinical Oncology, 2018, evaluating the role of stereotactic body RT (SBRT) in combination with PD1 blockade in a randomized fashion (see **Table 2**). Seventy-eight patients with advanced non-small-cell lung cancer (NSCLC) were randomized to receive pembrolizumab or pembrolizumab preceded by SBRT (24 Gy in 3 fractions) to a single metastatic site. Median progression-free survival (PFS) was 7.1 months in the SBRT arm versus 2.8 months in the pembrolizumab alone arm. With SBRT, the objective response rate (ORR) was increased from 21% to

39%.[23] In a separate study, 48 patients with M1 HNSCC were randomized to receive nivolumab 3 mg/kg q2 weeks with or without SBRT to a single lesion (59% lung lesions, 27 Gy in 3 fractions) between cycles 1 and 2 of nivolumab. In this study, the primary endpoint of ORR in non-irradiated lesions was not significantly different between the arms, 25.9% with SBRT and 30.8% without SBRT. Of interest, response rates were significantly higher in virus-negative (HPV-negative, EBV-negative patients) and in high mutational burden tumors.[24] In summary, despite anecdotal observations, higher level evidence for the abscopal effects is currently limited. Ongoing work seems promising in identifying subsets of patients who may benefit from improved outcomes with radiotherapy and ICB.

## SAFETY OF RADIOTHERAPY AND IMMUNE CHECKPOINT BLOCKADE IN THE CURATIVE TREATMENT SETTING

Combinations of immunotherapy and radiation delivered to many organs and tumor sites at palliative doses in the metastatic setting do not result in a substantial increase in adverse events, aside from a possible association with increased risk of radiation necrosis following cranial irradiation.[25] In the context of definitive treatment, however, the significance of possible compounded toxicity from RT and ICB combinations are of renewed importance, as adverse events may prevent patients from receiving appropriate curative therapy. Furthermore, radiation doses administered with definitive intent are higher than those used for palliative treatment, and radiation-associated toxicities are thus more prevalent. In addition, the risk of "hyperprogression," or rapid growth of tumor following initiation of therapy, has been reported in 9% to 17% of patients who undergo ICB for metastatic disease.[26–28] Although the mechanisms responsible for this phenomenon and predictors remain to be characterized, the possibility of introducing a risk of hyperprogression in the definitive setting with ICB is also a potential concern. Furthermore, as follow-up is limited from prospective trials, the long-term effects of ICB and combination therapy are not yet well characterized and will be of significant consequence for patients with curable disease and longer life expectancy than in metastatic populations. As such, the safety of definitive dose RT and ICB in the curative setting needs to be carefully assessed separately from studies conducted in patients with metastatic disease.

Current prospective trials evaluating ICB and radiotherapy in the definitive setting are summarized in **Table 1**. An early report from a phase Ib trial assessing safety of concurrent and adjuvant pembrolizumab administered with cisplatin-based radiotherapy found that pembrolizumab does not compromise delivery of full dose chemoradiation. Of 27 patients, all completed the full dose of radiation (70 Gy), and 23/27 (85%) received the target dose of cisplatin (>=200 mg/m$^2$). Twenty-one (78%) patients received all of the prescribed doses of pembrolizumab and only 3 discontinued because of immune-related adverse events (peripheral neuropathy, increased aspartate aminotransferase level, and Lhermitte-like syndrome).[29]

GORTEC 2015-01 is a phase II randomized trial comparing cetuximab-based chemoradiation with pembrolizumab-based radiation for definitive therapy of locally advanced HNSCC in cisplatin-ineligible patients. As of the most recent report, 133 patients were randomized; treatment compliance was high with 92% of patients receiving the prescribed radiotherapy dose of 69.96 Gy in 33 fractions and 87% of patients receiving the prescribed course of 3 administrations of pembrolizumab. Lower rates of grade 3+ adverse events were observed with pembrolizumab compared with cetuximab, including dermatitis (19% vs 59%), mucositis (31% vs 59%), and rash (0% vs 15%). Of note, higher rates of thyroiditis were noted with pembrolizumab (18% vs 6%).[30]

**Table 1**
Prospective safety data evaluating radiotherapy and immune checkpoint blockade combinations in the definitive setting

| Study | Cancer Histology | Population | Primary Endpoint(s) | Immune Checkpoint Inhibitor | ICB Dose/Schedule | Other Concurrent Systemic Therapy | Radiation Dose | Toxicity Data | Response Data |
|---|---|---|---|---|---|---|---|---|---|
| Powell et al,[29] ASCO 2017, NCT02586207 | Head and neck squamous cell carcinoma N = 27 safety cohort (expansion cohort N = 57 planned) | Cisplatin eligible stage III-IVB | Dose-limiting AEs CR rate at day 150 | Pembrolizumab anti-PD1 | 200 mg every 3 wk × 8 doses | Cisplatin 40 mg/m$^2$ × 6 doses | 70 Gy/35 fx | 3 ICB discontinuations due irAEs (AST elevation, peripheral motor neuropathy, Lhermitte-like syndrome) 44% grade 3 dysphagia 30% grade 3 mucositis 15% grade 3 radiation dermatitis 15% grade 3 weight loss | 78% with CR at day 150<br>• 85% for HPV+<br>• 57% for HPV− |
| RTOG 3504 Ferris et al,[42] ASCO 2018, Gillison et al,[43] IJROBP 2018, NCT02764593 | Head and neck squamous cell carcinoma N = 29 | Intermediate-high risk (based on stage, smoking history and p16 status) | DLT | Nivolumab anti-PD1 | 240 mg every 14 d × 10 concurrent (360 mg every 21 d for arm 2), 480 mg every 28 d × 7 adjuvant | Arm 1: cisplatin 40 mg/m$^2$ every wk × 7 doses Arm 2: cisplatin 100 mg/m$^2$ every 21 d × 3 doses Arm 3: cetuximab 250/400 mg/m$^2$ every wk × 7 doses | 70 Gy/35 fx | Arm 1: 0/10 DLT Arm 2: 0/10 DLT Arm 3: 1/9 DLT (grade 3 mucositis) | Arm 1: 0 events (median f/u 11.5 mo) Arm 2: 1 death (median f/u 10.4 mo) Arm 3: 1 disease progression (median f/u 8.0 mo) |
| GORTEC 2015-01 "PembroRad" Sun et al,[30] ASCO 2018, NCT02707588 | Head and neck squamous cell carcinoma N = 133 | Cisplatin ineligible stage III-IVB | Locoregional control at 15 mo | Pembrolizumab anti-PD1 | 200 mg every 3 wk during RT | Arm 1: Pembrolizumab-RT Arm 2: cetuximab-RT | 69.96 Gy/33 fx | Grade 3 + AEs (pembrolizumab vs cetuximab): dermatitis 19% vs 31% mucositis 59% vs 59% rash 0% vs 15% dysthyroidism 18% vs 6% | NA |

| Trial | Cancer | Setting | Endpoint | Agent | Dose | Comparator | RT dose | Toxicity | Response |
|---|---|---|---|---|---|---|---|---|---|
| GORTEC 2017-01 REACH trial Tao et al,[31] ASCO 2017, NCT02999087 | Head and neck squamous cell carcinoma N = 29 (total n = 688 planned) | High-dose cisplatin eligible of ineligible | PFS | Avelumab anti-PDL1 | 10 mg/kg every 2 wk | Cetuximab 400 mg/m² loading dose, 250 mg/m² weekly | 69.96 Gy/33 fx 7 wk IMRT | 3 patients with grade 4 AEs (dermatitis, lymphopenia, oral mucositis) | NA |
| Weiss et al,[32] ASCO 2018, NCT02609503 | Head and neck squamous cell carcinoma N = 16 (N = 29 planned) | Cisplatin ineligible stage III-IVA | PFS | Pembrolizumab anti-PD1 | 200 mg every 3 wk × 6 doses | NA | | Grade 3 AEs: 7 lymphopenia 5 mucositis 1 nausea 1 anorexia | NA |
| DUART trial, Joshi et al,[33] ASCO 2018, NCT02891161 | Bladder cancer N = 6 (n = 42 planned) | Unresectable or unfit for surgery, T3-4, N0-2, after neoadjuvant chemotherapy | Safety | Durvalumab anti-PDL1 | 1500 mg day 1, day 28 and adjuvantly every 4 wk for 12 mo | NA | 64.8 Gy/36 fx | No DLTs observed in the 5/6 patients that have completed durvalumab-RT, no grade 3 irAEs. Most common toxicity fatigue (3/6, 50%) | 3/4 patients with ongoing response after durvalumab-RT, 1 with progression |
| ETOP NICOLAS, Peters et al,[59] ASCO 2018, NCT02434081 | Non-small cell lung cancer (n = 58 safety cohort) | Stage III (N2/3) | Primary safety endpoint: grade 3 pneumonitis | Nivolumab anti-PD1 | 360 mg every 4 wk, followed by 480 mg every 4 wk for up to 1 y | Platinum based (with etoposide, vinorelbine or pemetrexed) | 66 Gy/33 fx | 13 grade 1/2 pneumonitis events (22.4%), 6 grade 3 pneumonitis events (10.3%), 3 grade 5 events (5.2%, 2 stroke, 1 esophageal fistula) | NA |

(continued on next page)

**Table 1**
*(continued)*

| Study | Cancer Histology | Population | Primary Endpoint(s) | Immune Checkpoint Inhibitor | ICB Dose/Schedule | Other Concurrent Systemic Therapy | Radiation Dose | Toxicity Data | Response Data |
|---|---|---|---|---|---|---|---|---|---|
| LUN 14-179, Durm et al,[40] ASCO 2018, NCT02343952 | Non-small cell lung cancer N = 93 | Stage III unresectable | Time to metastatic disease or death | Pembrolizumab anti-PD1 | 200 mg every 3 wk for up to 1 y (consolidation 4–8 wk after CRT if no progression) | NA | 59–66.6 Gy | Grade 3 + toxicities: Pneumonitis 6.5% Fatigue 4.3% Cough 1.1% Dyspnea 5.4% Diarrhea 4.3% Other 4.3% | Median time to metastatic disease or death: 22.4 mo Median PFS 17.0 mo Median OS: not reached 12 mo OS: 81.0% 24 mo OS: 61.9% |
| PACIFIC trial, Antonia et al,[38] 2017, NEJM, NCT02125461 | Non-small cell lung cancer N = 713 (2:1 randomization to receive durvalumab) | Stage III unresectable | PFS and OS | Durvalumab anti-PDL1 | 10 mg/kg every 2 wk for up to 12 mo (consolidation beginning 1–42 d after completion of RT) | NA | 54–66 Gy | Durvalumab vs placebo: Any grade 3–4: 29.9% vs 26.1% Pneumonitis: 3.4% vs 2.6% Grade 5 toxicity: 4.4% vs 5.6% Grade 5 pneumonitis: 0.8% vs 1.3% Dyspnea 1.5% vs 2.6% Pneumonia 4.4% vs 3.8% | Durvalumab vs placebo: Median time to death or distant metastasis: 23.2 vs 14.6 mo 18-mo PFS: 44.2% 27.0% |

*Abbreviations:* AEs, adverse events; ASCO, American Society of Clinical Oncology; CR, complete response; CRT, chemoradiation; DLT, dose-limiting toxicity; f/u, follow-up; irAEs, immune-related adverse events; NA, not applicable.

The REACH trial (GORTEC 2017-01) is a phase III trial randomizing patients with locally advanced HNSCC to receive standard of care cisplatin-RT or cetuximab-RT (if cisplatin ineligible) versus the experimental arm of cetuximab-RT with concurrent and adjuvant avelumab (anti-PDL1) for 12 months. Results from the lead-in phase of the protocol revealed that the experimental combination is reasonably well tolerated. Of 14 patients accrued, 3 patients (21.4%) developed grade 4 toxicities (dermatitis, mucositis, and lymphopenia).[31]

Preliminary toxicity data from a multi-center phase II trial of combination pembrolizumab with definitive dose radiation in cisplatin-ineligible patients were also recently reported (NCT02609503). All patients completed 70 Gy RT and 15/16 enrolled completed the 6 prescribed cycles of pembrolizumab. Seven cases of grade 3 + lymphopenia, 5 cases of grade 3 mucositis and 1 case each of grade 3 nausea and anorexia were observed. Three treatment failures have occurred thus far.[32]

The DUART trial (NCT02891161) is currently enrolling patients with locally advanced unresectable bladder cancer to receive induction chemotherapy followed by durvalumab (anti-PDL1) in combination with radiotherapy followed by adjuvant durvalumab. Early safety data from 6 patients showed that 5 of 6 were able to complete durvalumab-RT without dose-limiting toxicity with the most common adverse event being fatigue (50%). No grade 3 events have been observed thus far.[33]

## EFFICACY OF RADIOTHERAPY AND IMMUNE CHECKPOINT BLOCKADE IN THE CURATIVE TREATMENT SETTING

It is noteworthy that in many trials that showed superiority of immunotherapy, survival curves overlapped early and separated only later (as opposed to separating continuously over time, as would be expected by proportional hazards). A previous analysis of several landmark immunotherapy trials demonstrated significant deviation from proportional hazards in these trials and a more significant benefit from immunotherapy when the initial 20% of events are excluded.[34] These findings suggest that patients who have early disease progression may be less likely to benefit from immune checkpoint monotherapy. Although effects from cytotoxic therapies typically have a relatively rapid onset, the mechanism of action of most immunotherapies relies on the generation of an adaptive immune response and accumulation of immune effector cells over time. Consistent with this notion, the ratio of invigorated T cells to tumor burden has been demonstrated to predict response in melanoma patients treated with pembrolizumab.[35] In this way, patients with extensive disease and/or rapid progression may not derive as much benefit from immunotherapy combinations, and treatment may be discontinued early because of lack of perceived response. This is supported by the observation from a randomized trial of ipilimumab versus placebo following RT for bone metastases in metastatic castrate-resistant prostate cancer, in which patients with unfavorable features (alkaline phosphatase >1.5× upper limit of normal, hemoglobin <11 g/dL and presence of visceral metastasis)[36] derived less benefit compared with patients who did not have these features. Similarly, patients with high lactate dehydrogenase and liver metastases as a group have shorter overall survival (OS) following treatment with anti-CTLA4 or anti-PD1 therapy.[37] As previously mentioned, a subset of patients treated with ICB may experience hyperprogression; thus, there may be a rationale for irradiation of all locoregional disease before use of immunotherapies to potentially minimize this risk. Taken together, these findings highlight an additional role for radiation or other adjunct therapies to delay progression and potentially avoid discontinuation of ICB because of early progression, thus allowing immune responses to build up and reach their full effect. In addition, it provides further rationale for the use of immunotherapies for patients in the locally advanced or adjuvant setting, when there is limited disease burden and a higher likelihood of improved outcome.

## CLINICAL TRIALS TESTING RADIOTHERAPY AND IMMUNE CHECKPOINT BLOCKADE IN THE CURATIVE TREATMENT SETTING

The PACIFIC trial is a landmark study that assessed the benefit of adjuvant treatment with the anti-PDL1 antibody durvalumab in patients with stage III NSCLC after treatment with platinum-based definitive chemoradiotherapy. Patients (713) were randomized in a 2:1 ratio to receive durvalumab or placebo for up to 12 months. The median time to death or distant metastasis was extended significantly in the group receiving durvalumab (14.6 vs 23.2 months) with an 18-month PFS rate of 44.2% versus 27.0%.[38] Virtually all subgroups of patients demonstrated clinical benefit from durvalumab, even patients with minimal tumor PDL1 expression. In a recent planned interim analysis, the trial had met its second of 2 primary endpoints with durvalumab showing a statistically significant benefit in OS compared with placebo.[39] Thus, this study provides some of the first randomized evidence for the significant clinical benefit of immunotherapy in the locally advanced setting when used in sequenced combination with definitive radiation.

A similar trial assessing the role of adjuvant nivolumab in stage III NSCLC recently reported early efficacy results comparable with those of the PACIFIC trial. In 93 patients who had not progressed 4 to 8 weeks after definitive platinum-based chemoradiation for stage III disease and received nivolumab for up to 1 year, the median time to metastatic disease or death was 22.4 months, with a median PFS of 17.0 months and median OS not reached. Of note, only 6.5% of patients experienced grade 3+ pneumonitis.[40]

As further evidence of the potentiating effect of radiotherapy to ICB, retrospective subset analyses in the KEYNOTE-001 trial for patients with progressive locally advanced or metastatic NSCLC, revealed that patients who had undergone prior treatment with radiotherapy experienced significantly longer PFS (hazard ratio [HR], 0.56; median PFS, 4.4 vs 2.1 months) and longer OS (HR, 0.58; OS, 11.6 vs 5.3 months).[41] These data, in combination with the above-described prospective data, including the PACIFIC trial, strongly suggest that consolidative ICB is an effective strategy in the locally advanced setting following definitive radiotherapy-based treatment.

There are multiple ongoing trials assessing the role of ICB in the definitive treatment of locally advanced HSNCC. RTOG 3504 is evaluating the safety of combining concurrent and adjuvant nivolumab with cisplatin and cetuximab-based chemoradiation for patients with intermediate or high-risk locoregionally advanced HSNCC. Patients on this study receive nivolumab with either weekly cisplatin-based chemo-RT, bolus cisplatin-based chemo-RT, cetuximab-RT, or RT without other systemic therapy if cisplatin ineligible. Whereas the primary endpoint of the study is dose-limiting grade 3+ toxicity, early efficacy data are promising. At a median follow-up of 11.5 months in the weekly cisplatin arm (n = 10), no deaths or disease progression events have been observed. Of the 9 patients in the bolus cisplatin arm, only 1 death and disease progression events have been observed, and in the cetuximab arm, 1 disease progression event and no deaths have been observed.[42,43]

A retrospective analysis of patients with brain metastases from NSCLC, renal cell carcinoma, or melanoma treated with radiotherapy to the brain in combination with anti-PD1 therapy from 4 centers demonstrated favorable clinical outcomes compared with historical controls, with a median survival of 634 days after initiation of brain radiation. Furthermore, of 59 patients who started brain radiation after initiation anti-PD1 therapy, the 25 who continued to receive anti-PD1 therapy demonstrated improved survival.[44] Multiple other reports have also demonstrated favorable outcomes in patients treated with anti-CTLA-4 or anti-PD1 therapy and brain radiation.[45,46]

Considerations of how to best design the radiation field when combining radiotherapy with immunotherapy may also be important. In particular, irradiation of draining lymphatic basins on an elective basis, which is done routinely in many settings including locally advanced HSNCC, may have an impact on immune cell trafficking and immunomodulatory response. A preclinical model of irradiation of tumor ± tumor-draining lymph nodes with ICB demonstrated a reduction in adaptive immune responses with elective nodal radiation resulting in a reduction in chemokine expression and reduced immune infiltration that negatively impacted survival.[47] Specifically, following irradiation of lymph nodes in addition to tumor, lower density of intratumoral effector T cells was observed, lower concentrations of IFN-γ and TNF-α were seen, and there was noted to be attenuation of production of chemokines, including CSCL10, CCL3, and CCL5, that are known to play a role in CD8+ T cell recruitment. In locally advanced lung cancer, radiation targets are typically limited to sites of tumor and involved nodal stations without irradiation of significant volumes of uninvolved draining lymphatics, which may be another reason why such a robust response was seen in the PACIFIC trial.[38]

## IDEAL TIMING AND SEQUENCING OF RADIATION AND IMMUNE CHECKPOINT BLOCKADE

The question of optimal timing of ICB relative to radiotherapy is an important and practical one that may have significant bearing on the efficacy of combined approaches. Specifically, it remains unknown whether a synergistic effect is best achieved with ICB delivered before, during, or following radiation. If the timing or sequence is suboptimal, the potential immunosuppressive effects of RT may theoretically hinder the systemic response of ICB. In addition, relative timing may have important implications not just for efficacy but also for safety and tolerability.

Clinically, most case reports that have identified an abscopal effect with RT + ICB combinations have found it to occur when RT was given concurrently or immediately following ICB. This is consistent with the notion that ICB may prime the immune system to recognize radiation-induced antigen release and presentation. A retrospective analysis of 750 patients treated at the Memorial Sloan Kettering Cancer Center, who received radiation and ICB (anti-CTLA4 or anti-PD1/PDL1), found that median OS was improved when patients received RT concurrently with ICB (20 months) compared with those who received ICB first (6 months) or RT first (7 months).[48] In addition, patients who received ICB for a period of greater than 30 days before RT also experienced improved survival, again suggesting a benefit to immune priming before RT. This is corroborated by a report of 75 melanoma patients with brain metastases who underwent stereotactic radiosurgery and ICB. Patients who received therapy concomitantly (RT within 4 weeks of ICB) experienced more dramatic reduction in lesion size at 1.5, 3, and 6 months following RT.[46] The importance of timing was also suggested in an analysis of the PACIFIC trial, which demonstrated that patients who were randomized to start durvalumab within 14 days of the completion of RT experienced improved PFS compared with those who started durvalumab 14 to 42 days after RT (HR for progression or death 0.39 vs 0.63).[38] In preclinical models, the efficacy of administering 10 Gy in 2 fractions was enhanced when anti-PDL1 antibody was delivered concurrently at the beginning of RT (day 1) or at the end of RT (day 5), but not when given sequentially 7 days following completion of RT.[15]

Nevertheless, optimal timing may be dependent on multiple mitigating factors including radiation dose, fractionation, as well as the ICB target. Tumor-bearing mice treated with a single high dose of radiotherapy (20 Gy) were found to have differing optimal timings of ICB dependent on whether they received anti-CTLA4 or anti-OX40 antibodies. With CTLA4 blockade, maximum efficacy was found when given before radiation, potentially owing to depletion of regulatory T cells; with anti-OX40, the optimal time point was found to be 1 day following radiation presumably because of maximal antigen presentation.[49]

The ideal timing and sequencing of therapies is currently being explored in prospective clinical trials. UPCI 15-132 (NCT02777385) randomizes patients with locally advanced HNSCC to receive pembrolizumab as adjuvant therapy (beginning 3 weeks after RT) or concurrently (given 1 week before and during RT). The DETERRED trial at MD Anderson is an ongoing study for patients receiving definitive chemoradiation for non-metastatic NSCLC that is comparing the use of atezolizumab (anti-PDL1) given as adjuvant therapy versus concurrently with radiotherapy and then as adjuvant therapy (NCT02525757).

## OPTIMAL RADIOTHERAPY DOSAGE AND FRACTIONATION

Depending on the disease and context, RT can be delivered to a wide range of doses and fractionation schemes from conventionally fractionated radiation (1.8–2 Gy per fraction) to moderately hypofractionated schedules (2–6 Gy per fraction) to high-dose single-fraction treatment. It is likely that mechanisms of radiation-induced cell death differ depending on the dose per fraction that is used. However, classical dose and fractionation schedules may need to be reconsidered when defining optimal synergy with immunomodulating agents as the goal of therapy is different. In theory, prolonged fractionation may hamper the radiation-induced immune response by continually eradicating immune cell fractions infiltrating the tumor or draining nodal basins,[47] which are known to be highly radiosensitive.

Camphausen and colleagues[50] developed a mouse model of the abscopal effect by assessing Lewis lung carcinoma or T241 fibrosarcoma tumor growth in the midline dorsum following separate irradiation of the animal's leg. Comparing regimens of 50 Gy in 5 fractions versus 24 Gy in 12 fractions, the higher dose per fraction treatment resulted in improved abscopal tumor growth inhibition in a p53-dependent fashion. In a mouse model of melanoma, anti-tumor immune responses were assessed following irradiation with 15 Gy in a single fraction versus 15 Gy in 5 fractions. Single-fraction irradiation was associated with an increase in immune activation in draining lymphatics as well as an increase in IFN-$\gamma$-secreting tumor-infiltrating lymphocytes and cytoloysis.[5] In a separate preclinical study, treatment with 20 Gy in a single fraction was found to be more effective than 20 Gy delivered in 4 fractions and, interestingly, the enhancement in efficacy was reversed with administration of anti-CD8 antibody, suggesting a critical role for cytotoxic T cells following treatment with high-dose single-fraction radiation.[4] Fractionated radiotherapy, it was hypothesized, may eradicate tumor-directed effector T cells over the course of treatment.

These studies have therefore demonstrated a rationale for the use of hypofractionated or large dose per fraction treatment to enhance anti-tumor immune responses and promote an abscopal effect. In the clinical setting, this has also been corroborated by a retrospective review of patients treated with radiotherapy and ICB, which found that treatment with hypofractionated radiation (>4 Gy per fraction) was associated with longer OS.[48] However, prospective studies are needed to define the benefit of adding hypofractionated radiotherapy or SBRT to ICB (**Table 2**).

Still, the question of whether conventionally fractionated versus hypofractionated or high- versus low-dose radiation is most suitable remains unanswered. Although the above data point toward SBRT doses being most effective, it has also been demonstrated that fractionated radiation, albeit still hypofractionated, was more effective at mediating an abscopal effect than single high-dose treatment (24 Gy in 3 fractions or 30 Gy in 5 fractions compared with 20–30 Gy in 1 fraction) when combined with anti-CTLA4 blockade.[11,51] Single-fraction doses in the 20–30-Gy range inhibit cGAS-STING activation and may therefore be less likely to elicit the necessary cytosolic DNA immunogenic response.[51] A separate preclinical model also demonstrated that fractionated RT (10 Gy in 10 fractions compared with 1 fraction) was more effective at activating cellular immune response expression profiles and release of pro-inflammatory damage-associated molecular pattern molecules.[52]

At the present time, no prospective clinical data exist to define the optimal radiation dose for induction of an abscopal effect. Low-dose radiation (<1 Gy per fraction) may have significant clinically relevant immunologic effects.[53] Ongoing trials are randomizing patients to receive high- versus low-dose radiation in combination with checkpoint blockade in HNSCC, NSCLC and colorectal cancer (NCT03085719, ETCTN 10021).

## FUTURE DIRECTIONS

Although the vast majority of data regarding radiotherapy combined with immune modulation exist in the context of PD1/PDL1 or CTLA4 blockade, multiple other immune checkpoints and targets are currently being prospectively evaluated, including OX40, TIM3, GITR, and LAG3.[54] How these agents will work in concert with radiotherapy remains to be seen. In addition, combinatorial effects with radiotherapy are also being explored with other forms of immunotherapy, such as high-dose interleukin-2 with or without SBRT in melanoma patients (NCT01416831), which has demonstrated promising results in phase 1 studies.[55] In early preclinical studies, radiotherapy has also been found to sensitize tumor cells to chimeric antigen receptor T cells,[56] which have resulted in profound effects in hematologic malignancies. In light of the improved understanding of the molecular mechanisms underlying the abscopal effect, delivery of pharmacologic adjuvants, such as STING agonists, may also potentiate systemic immune responses induced with radiotherapy.[9,10,51]

Whereas radiotherapy is typically administered to the entirety of the gross tumor volume, there are theoretic detrimental immunosuppressive effects to irradiating surrounding-infiltrating lymphocytes. As an experimental approach, partial tumor irradiation may be sufficient for treatment of some tumors,[57,58] the added benefit being of the sparing of adjacent normal tissue of toxicity and perhaps allowing an infiltrating immune response to proceed unhampered. The use of more conformal radiotherapy techniques, such as brachytherapy, proton therapy, or other particle therapy, to reduce irradiation of surrounding tissues also remains to be explored in this context.

The potential benefits of combining radiotherapy with immunotherapies, particularly ICB, are supported by robust preclinical evidence demonstrating synergy. Broadly, these combinations seem to be safe, with few reports to date of undue toxicity, even when radiotherapy is administered at definitive doses. The outcomes reported with the use of ICB following definitive chemoradiation in the PACIFIC trial represent the greatest magnitude of benefit demonstrated for immunotherapy in NSCLC, further

**Table 2**
Randomized prospective trials evaluating abscopal effects from combining immune checkpoint blockade with radiotherapy

| Study | Cancer Histology/ Population | Primary Endpoint | Immune Checkpoint Inhibitor | ICB Dose/ Schedule | Radiotherapy Regimen | Response Data |
|---|---|---|---|---|---|---|
| McBride et al,[24] ASCO 2018, NCT02684253 | Metastatic HNSCC N = 53 | ORR in unirradiated lesions | Nivolumab anti-PD1 | 3 mg/kg every 2 wk | 27 Gy in 3 fractions (SBRT) delivered between cycles 1 and 2 of nivolumab | Nivolumab vs Nivolumab + SBRT: ORR: 30.8% vs 25.9%, $P = .93$ (trend toward improved ORR with SBRT and nivolumab in virus-negative cohort) 1-y PFS: 28% vs 16%, $P = .89$ 1-y OS: 46% vs 54%, $P = .46$ |
| "PEMBRO-RT," Theelen et al,[23] ASCO 2018 | Advanced NSCLC (second line or more treatment) N = 74 | ORR | Pembrolizumab anti-PD1 | 200 mg every 3 wk | 24 Gy in 3 fractions (SBRT) delivered within 7 d before first cycle of pembrolizumab | Pembrolizumab vs Pembrolizumab + SBRT: ORR at 12 wk: 21% vs 39%, $P = .28$ (more responders in PDL1-negative group with SBRT) Median PFS: 2.8 mo vs 7.1 mo, $P = .08$ Median OS: 7.6 mo vs 19.2 mo, $P = .1$ |

*Abbreviation:* AST, aspartate aminotransferase.

heightening interest in combining radiotherapy and immunotherapy. Ongoing and future studies will characterize the optimal patient subsets, immunotherapy agents, radiation dosages, and targets, as well as the sequence of therapies to maximize the safety and efficacy of this promising combinatorial approach.

## REFERENCES

1. Chera BS, Amdur RJ, Mendenhall W, et al. Beware of deintensification of radiation therapy in patients with p16-positive oropharynx cancer and rheumatological diseases. Pract Radiat Oncol 2017;7(4):e261–2.
2. Stone HB, Peters LJ, Milas L. Effect of host immune capability on radiocurability and subsequent transplantability of a murine fibrosarcoma. J Natl Cancer Inst 1979;63(5):1229–35.
3. Spanos WC, Nowicki P, Lee DW, et al. Immune response during therapy with cisplatin or radiation for human papillomavirus-related head and neck cancer. Arch Otolaryngol Head Neck Surg 2009;135(11):1137–46.
4. Lee Y, Auh SL, Wang Y, et al. Therapeutic effects of ablative radiation on local tumor require CD8+ T cells: changing strategies for cancer treatment. Blood 2009; 114(3):589–95.
5. Lugade AA, Moran JP, Gerber SA, et al. Local radiation therapy of B16 melanoma tumors increases the generation of tumor antigen-specific effector cells that traffic to the tumor. J Immunol 2005;174(12):7516–23.
6. Apetoh L, Ghiringhelli F, Tesniere A, et al. Toll-like receptor 4-dependent contribution of the immune system to anticancer chemotherapy and radiotherapy. Nat Med 2007;13(9):1050–9.
7. Burnette BC, Liang H, Lee Y, et al. The efficacy of radiotherapy relies upon induction of type I interferon-dependent innate and adaptive immunity. Cancer Res 2011;71(7):2488–96.
8. Reits EA, Hodge JW, Herberts CA, et al. Radiation modulates the peptide repertoire, enhances MHC class I expression, and induces successful antitumor immunotherapy. J Exp Med 2006;203(5):1259–71.
9. Deng L, Liang H, Xu M, et al. STING-dependent cytosolic DNA sensing promotes radiation-induced type I interferon-dependent antitumor immunity in immunogenic tumors. Immunity 2014;41(5):843–52.
10. Woo S-R, Fuertes MB, Corrales L, et al. STING-dependent cytosolic DNA sensing mediates innate immune recognition of immunogenic tumors. Immunity 2014; 41(5):830–42.
11. Dewan MZ, Galloway AE, Kawashima N, et al. Fractionated but not single-dose radiotherapy induces an immune-mediated abscopal effect when combined with anti-CTLA-4 antibody. Clin Cancer Res 2009;15(17):5379–88.
12. Demaria S, Kawashima N, Yang AM, et al. Immune-mediated inhibition of metastases after treatment with local radiation and CTLA-4 blockade in a mouse model of breast cancer. Clin Cancer Res 2005;11(2 Pt 1):728–34.
13. Zeng J, See AP, Phallen J, et al. Anti-PD-1 blockade and stereotactic radiation produce long-term survival in mice with intracranial gliomas. Int J Radiat Oncol Biol Phys 2013;86(2):343–9.
14. Deng L, Liang H, Burnette B, et al. Irradiation and anti-PD-L1 treatment synergistically promote antitumor immunity in mice. J Clin Invest 2014;124(2):687–95.
15. Dovedi SJ, Adlard AL, Lipowska-Bhalla G, et al. Acquired resistance to fractionated radiotherapy can be overcome by concurrent PD-L1 blockade. Cancer Res 2014;74(19):5458–68.

16. Sharabi AB, Nirschl CJ, Kochel CM, et al. Stereotactic radiation therapy augments antigen-specific PD-1-mediated antitumor immune responses via cross-presentation of tumor antigen. Cancer Immunol Res 2015;3(4):345–55.

17. Twyman-Saint Victor C, Rech AJ, Maity A, et al. Radiation and dual checkpoint blockade activate non-redundant immune mechanisms in cancer. Nature 2015; 520(7547):373–7.

18. Abuodeh Y, Venkat P, Kim S. Systematic review of case reports on the abscopal effect. Curr Probl Cancer 2016;40(1):25–37.

19. Postow MA, Callahan MK, Barker CA, et al. Immunologic correlates of the abscopal effect in a patient with melanoma. N Engl J Med 2012;366(10):925–31.

20. Hiniker SM, Chen DS, Reddy S, et al. A systemic complete response of metastatic melanoma to local radiation and immunotherapy. Transl Oncol 2012;5(6): 404–7.

21. Stamell EF, Wolchok JD, Gnjatic S, et al. The abscopal effect associated with a systemic anti-melanoma immune response. Int J Radiat Oncol Biol Phys 2013; 85(2):293–5.

22. Golden EB, Demaria S, Schiff PB, et al. An abscopal response to radiation and ipilimumab in a patient with metastatic non-small cell lung cancer. Cancer Immunol Res 2013;1(6):365–72.

23. Theelen W, Peulen@Nki H, NI NF, et al. Randomized phase II study of pembrolizumab after stereotactic body radiotherapy (SBRT) versus pembrolizumab alone in patients with advanced non-small cell lung cancer: the PEMBRO-RT study. J Clin Oncol 2018;36(15_suppl):9023.

24. McBride SM, Sherman EJ, Tsai CJ, et al. A phase II randomized trial of nivolumab with stereotactic body radiotherapy (SBRT) versus nivolumab alone in metastatic (M1) head and neck squamous cell carcinoma (HNSCC). J Clin Oncol 2018; 36(15_suppl):6009.

25. Hwang WL, Pike LRG, Royce TJ, et al. Safety of combining radiotherapy with immune-checkpoint inhibition. Nat Rev Clin Oncol 2018;15(8):477–94.

26. Champiat S, Dercle L, Ammari S, et al. Hyperprogressive disease is a new pattern of progression in cancer patients treated by anti-PD-1/PD-L1. Clin Cancer Res 2017;23(8):1920–8.

27. Kato S, Goodman A, Walavalkar V, et al. Hyperprogressors after immunotherapy: analysis of genomic alterations associated with accelerated growth rate. Clin Cancer Res 2017;23(15):4242–50.

28. Kim Y, Kim CH, Kim HS, et al. Hyperprogression after immunotherapy: clinical implication and genomic alterations in advanced non-small cell lung cancer patients (NSCLC). J Clin Oncol 2018;36(15_suppl):9075.

29. Powell SF, Gitau MM, Sumey CJ, et al. Safety of pembrolizumab with chemoradiation (CRT) in locally advanced squamous cell carcinoma of the head and neck (LA-SCCHN). J Clin Oncol 2017;35(15_suppl):6011.

30. Sun XS, Sire C, Tao Y, et al. A phase II randomized trial of pembrolizumab versus cetuximab, concomitant with radiotherapy (RT) in locally advanced (LA) squamous cell carcinoma of the head and neck (SCCHN): first results of the GORTEC 2015-01 "PembroRad" trial. J Clin Oncol 2018;36(15_suppl):6018.

31. Tao Y, Auperin A, Sun XS, et al. Avelumab-cetuximab-radiotherapy (RT) versus standards of care (SoC) in locally advanced squamous cell carcinoma of the head and neck (SCCHN): safety phase of the randomized trial GORTEC 2017-01 (REACH). J Clin Oncol 2018;36(15_suppl):6076.

32. Weiss J, Bauman JR, Deal AM, et al. Preliminary toxicity data from the combination of pembrolizumab and definitive-dose radiotherapy for locally advanced

head and neck cancer with contraindication to cisplatin therapy. J Clin Oncol 2018;36(15_suppl):6069.

33. Joshi M, Tuanquin L, Kaag M, et al. Phase Ib study of concurrent durvalumab and radiation therapy (DUART) followed by adjuvant durvalumab in patients with urothelial cancer of the bladder: BTCRC-GU15-023 study. J Clin Oncol 2018; 36(6_suppl):455.

34. Alexander BM, Schoenfeld JD, Trippa L. Hazards of hazard ratios - deviations from model assumptions in immunotherapy. N Engl J Med 2018;378(12):1158–9.

35. Huang AC, Postow MA, Orlowski RJ, et al. T-cell invigoration to tumour burden ratio associated with anti-PD-1 response. Nature 2017;545(7652):60–5.

36. Kwon ED, Drake CG, Scher HI, et al. Ipilimumab versus placebo after radiotherapy in patients with metastatic castration-resistant prostate cancer that had progressed after docetaxel chemotherapy (CA184-043): a multicentre, randomised, double-blind, phase 3 trial. Lancet Oncol 2014;15(7):700–12.

37. Sen S, Hess K, Hong DS, et al. Development of a prognostic scoring system for patients with advanced cancer enrolled in immune checkpoint inhibitor phase 1 clinical trials. Br J Cancer 2018;118(6):763–9.

38. Antonia SJ, Villegas A, Daniel D, et al. Durvalumab after chemoradiotherapy in stage III non-small-cell lung cancer. N Engl J Med 2017;377(20):1919–29.

39. Imfinzi significantly improves overall survival in the Phase III PACIFIC trial for unresectable Stage III non-small cell lung cancer. Available at: https://www.astrazeneca.com/media-centre/press-releases/2018/imfinzi-significantly-improves-overall-survival-in-the-phase-iii-pacific-trial-for-unresectable-stage-iii-non-small-cell-lung-cancer-25052018.html. Accessed August 31, 2018.

40. Durm GA, Althouse SK, Sadiq AA, et al. Phase II trial of concurrent chemoradiation with consolidation pembrolizumab in patients with unresectable stage III non-small cell lung cancer: Hoosier Cancer Research Network LUN 14-179. J Clin Oncol 2018;36(15_suppl):8500.

41. Shaverdian N, Lisberg AE, Bornazyan K, et al. Previous radiotherapy and the clinical activity and toxicity of pembrolizumab in the treatment of non-small-cell lung cancer: a secondary analysis of the KEYNOTE-001 phase 1 trial. Lancet Oncol 2017;18(7):895–903.

42. Ferris RL, Gillison ML, Harris J, et al. Safety evaluation of nivolumab (Nivo) concomitant with cetuximab-radiotherapy for intermediate (IR) and high-risk (HR) local-regionally advanced head and neck squamous cell carcinoma (HNSCC): RTOG 3504. J Clin Oncol 2018;36(15_suppl):6010.

43. Gillison M, Ferris RL, Zhang Q, et al. Safety evaluation of nivolumab concomitant with platinum-based chemoradiation therapy for intermediate and high-risk local-regionally advanced head and neck squamous cell carcinoma: RTOG Foundation 3504. Int J Radiat Oncol Biol Phys 2018;100(5):1307–8.

44. Pike LRG, Bang A, Ott P, et al. Radiation and PD-1 inhibition: favorable outcomes after brain-directed radiation. Radiother Oncol 2017;124(1):98–103.

45. Ahmed KA, Stallworth DG, Kim Y, et al. Clinical outcomes of melanoma brain metastases treated with stereotactic radiation and anti-PD-1 therapy. Ann Oncol 2016;27(3):434–41.

46. Qian JM, Yu JB, Kluger HM, et al. Timing and type of immune checkpoint therapy affect the early radiographic response of melanoma brain metastases to stereotactic radiosurgery. Cancer 2016;122(19):3051–8.

47. Marciscano AE, Ghasemzadeh A, Nirschl TR, et al. Elective nodal irradiation attenuates the combinatorial efficacy of stereotactic radiation therapy and immunotherapy. Clin Cancer Res 2018. https://doi.org/10.1158/1078-0432.CCR-17-3427.

48. Samstein R, Rimner A, Barker CA, et al. Combined immune checkpoint blockade and radiation therapy: timing and dose fractionation associated with greatest survival duration among over 750 treated patients. Int J Radiat Oncol Biol Phys 2017; 99(2):S129–30.
49. Young KH, Baird JR, Savage T, et al. Optimizing timing of immunotherapy improves control of tumors by hypofractionated radiation therapy. PLoS One 2016;11(6):e0157164.
50. Camphausen K, Moses MA, Ménard C, et al. Radiation abscopal antitumor effect is mediated through p53. Cancer Res 2003;63(8):1990–3.
51. Vanpouille-Box C, Diamond JM, Pilones KA, et al. TGFβ is a master regulator of radiation therapy-induced antitumor immunity. Cancer Res 2015;75(11):2232–42.
52. John-Aryankalayil M, Palayoor ST, Cerna D, et al. Fractionated radiation therapy can induce a molecular profile for therapeutic targeting. Radiat Res 2010;174(4): 446–58.
53. Monjazeb AM, Schoenfeld JD. Radiation dose and checkpoint blockade immunotherapy: unanswered questions. Lancet Oncol 2016;17(1):e3–4.
54. Mahoney KM, Rennert PD, Freeman GJ. Combination cancer immunotherapy and new immunomodulatory targets. Nat Rev Drug Discov 2015;14(8):561–84.
55. Seung SK, Curti BD, Crittenden M, et al. Phase 1 study of stereotactic body radiotherapy and interleukin-2 – tumor and immunological responses. Sci Transl Med 2012;4(137):137ra74.
56. DeSelm CJ, Hamieh M, Sadelain M. Radiation sensitizes tumor cells to CAR T cell immunotherapy. Int J Radiat Oncol Biol Phys 2016;96(2):S127.
57. Samstein R, Markovsky E, Li H, et al. Partial tumor irradiation in a murine model is sufficient for tumor control via activation of an antitumor immune response. Int J Radiat Oncol Biol Phys 2017;99(2):E616–7.
58. Lemons JM, Luke JJ, Janisch L, et al. The ADscopal effect? control of partially irradiated versus completely irradiated tumors on a prospective trial of pembrolizumab and SBRT Per NRG-BR001. Int J Radiat Oncol Biol Phys 2017;99(2):S87.
59. Peters S, De Ruysscher D, Dafni U, et al. Safety evaluation of nivolumab added concurrently to radiotherapy in a standard first line chemo-RT regimen in unresectable locally advanced NSCLC: the ETOP NICOLAS phase II trial. J Clin Oncol 2018;36(15_suppl):8510.

# Intralesional Cancer Immunotherapies

Patrick A. Ott, MD, PhD[a,b,c,d,*]

## KEYWORDS

- Intralesional cancer immunotherapies • Oncolytic viral therapy
- Toll-like receptor agonists • STING agonists

## KEY POINTS

- Intralesional therapies are an attractive therapeutic strategy to induce T-cell inflammation in tumors.
- Various approaches, including oncolytic viral therapy, Toll-like receptor agonists, cytokines, and stimulator of interferon genes agonists, among others, are in clinical development.
- Talimogene laherparepvec is approved by regulatory agency for the treatment of advanced melanoma and has shown promise as partnering therapy with immune checkpoint inhibitors.

Effective tumor eradication by a host's immune response requires infiltration of the tumor with T cells that are specific and functional. As outlined in the cancer immunity cycle, these tumor-specific T cells are primed by dendritic cells (DCs) that capture tumor antigens in the tumor, process these antigens, and migrate to the tumor-draining lymph node, where they present them to T cells in the context of activation signals.[1] Batf3 DCs have been identified as a key DC subset that is able to cross-present tumor antigens through the class I major histocompatibility complex (MHC). Activation of Batf3 DCs, for example, through the stimulator of interferon genes (STING) pathway, induces a type I interferon (IFN) response, which is critical for T cell priming against tumor antigens. The presence of a CD8+ T-cell infiltrate in pretreatment tumor specimens from melanoma patients who received immune checkpoint inhibitor (ICI) therapy was associated with objective responses,[2,3] whereas patients with absent CD8+ T cells in pretreatment tumors were unlikely to respond. Up-regulation of

<sup>a</sup> Department of Medical Oncology, Melanoma Center, Center for Immuno-Oncology, Dana-Farber Cancer Institute, Harvard Medical School, 450 Brookline Avenue, Boston, MA 02215-5450, USA; <sup>b</sup> Department of Medicine, Brigham and Women's Hospital, Harvard Medical School, Boston, MA, USA; <sup>c</sup> Broad Institute of MIT and Harvard, Cambridge, MA, USA; <sup>d</sup> Harvard Medical School, Boston, MA, USA
* Melanoma Center, Center for Immuno-Oncology, Dana-Farber Cancer Institute, 450 Brookline Avenue, Boston, MA 02215-5450.
E-mail address: Patrick_Ott@DFCI.harvard.edu

Hematol Oncol Clin N Am 33 (2019) 249–260
https://doi.org/10.1016/j.hoc.2018.12.009
0889-8588/19/© 2018 Elsevier Inc. All rights reserved.

Programmed Death-Ligand 1 (PD-L1) in melanoma specimens has been linked to the presence of tumor-infiltrating lymphocytes and IFN-γ production (adaptive immune resistance), suggesting that PD-L1 in the tumor, also shown to be correlated with clinical benefit from ICI, is, at least in part, a surrogate marker for a T-cell inflamed tumor. Furthermore, gene expression profiling of pretreatment tumor biopsies has linked an inflamed signature reflecting up-regulation of type I IFNs, cytotoxic effector molecules, T-cell attracting chemokines, and antigen presentation to improved outcome both prognostically and in the context of immunotherapy.[4,5] Given that a vast majority of human cancers are not infiltrated by T cells at baseline, it does not seem surprising that objective response rates (ORRs) with ICI monotherapy generally do not exceed 20% to 30% in most tumor types whereas several common malignancies, including microsatellite stable colon cancer, pancreatic cancer, and prostate cancer are largely unresponsive to ICI. Although the mechanistic basis of absent tumor T-cell infiltration in a given patient is largely unknown, preclinical studies have implicated alterations in oncogenic signaling pathways including WNT-β-catenin, MYC, PTEN, and the p53 pathway as potentially causative factors of a non–T-cell inflamed tumor microenvironment.[6]

From a therapeutic perspective, given that the absence of an innate immune response is a defining element of the non–T-cell inflamed tumor microenvironment phenotype, a plausible approach to overcoming this phenotype is to directly induce this inflammatory response, thereby triggering the initial stimulus for the cascade of events that eventually leads to an effective immune response.

Intralesional cancer therapies are aimed at delivering such an inflammatory stimulus. Approaches that have already entered the clinic, including oncolytic viral therapy, agonists of Toll-like receptors (TLRs) and the STING pathway, and cytokines, are reviewed in this article.

## INTRALESIONAL ONCOLYTIC VIRAL THERAPY

Oncolytic viruses mediate antitumor immunity through various mechanisms (**Fig. 1**).

### Talimogene Laherparepvec

Talimogene laherparepvec (T-VEC) is an intratumorally administered oncolytic viral immunotherapy that is approved by the US Food and Drug Administration for the treatment of unresectable stage III and stage IV melanoma. The agent consists of a genetically engineered attenuated herpes simplex virus type 1; due to functional deletion of the infected cell protein 34.5, on injection into a tumor it replicates in cancer cells but not in normal tissue cells.[7] Insertion of the gene coding for granulocyte macrophage–colony stimulating factor (GM-CSF), a proinflammatory cytokine that mediates recruitment of DCs and macrophages into the tumor site and promotes maturation of DCs into effective antigen-presenting cells that can prime and activate tumor-specific T cells. Similar to other oncolytic viral therapies, T-VEC has 2 modes of action: (1) direct cytolysis of cancer cells and (2) an in situ vaccine effect mediated by release of tumor antigens that are cross-presented on the DCs attracted by GM-CSF. The vaccine effect creates systemic antitumor activity, which was initially seen in mouse studies (where it was dependent on GM-CSF expression [ie, not seen with T-VEC alone]) and has since been confirmed in human patients.

### Talimogene laherparepvec in melanoma: monotherapy

Clinically, T-VEC has been developed mainly in melanoma patients. Phase 1 and phase 2 studies demonstrated that the drug is overall well tolerated. The most common adverse events (AEs) related to T-VEC were local injection site reactions,

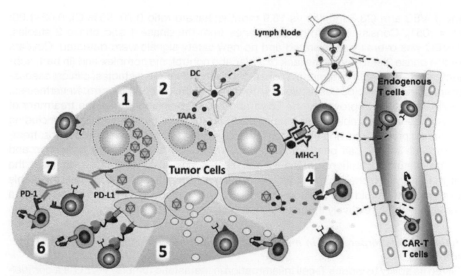

**Fig. 1.** Mechanisms by which OVs can mediate T-cell inflammation in the tumor: (1) direct oncolysis of tumor cells and increased tumor accessibility by creating space within the tumor mass; (2) release of damage-associated molecular patterns, PAMPs, and TAAs on tumor cell lysis that can recruit antigen presenting cells, and TAAs can be processed and presented to T cells at lymph node; (3) oncolytic virus infection can induce expression of MHC-I and β2-microblobulin; (4) oncolytic viruses can be engineered to express chemokines to increase infiltration of tumor-specific T cells; and (5) express inflammatory cytokines to increase T-cell priming at the tumor site. TAA, tumor-associated antigens; CAR-T cells, chimeric antigen receptor-T cells. (*From* Rosewell Shaw A, Suzuki M. Oncolytic viruses partner with T-cell therapy for solid tumor treatment. Front Immunol 2018;9:2103; with permission.)

constitutional symptoms, and nausea. Regression of both injected and noninjected metastases was seen in 6 of 26 evaluable patients with melanoma and other solid tumors in the phase 1 study[8] and in 13 of 50 melanoma patients in the phase 2 study,[9] which led to a phase 3 trial (OPTiM).[10] In this study, 436 patients with stage IIIB/C or stage IV melanoma were randomized 2:1 to receive either intratumoral injections of T-VEC or subcutaneous GM-CSF. GM-CSF as comparator arm was chosen based on historical data demonstrating improved overall survival in patients with high risk melanoma who received GM-CSF. The primary endpoint of the study was durable response rate, defined as a complete response (CR) or partial response (PR) lasting for 6 months or longer. T-VEC was given until CR, clinically significant progressive disease, intolerable toxicity, or 12 months of therapy not leading to an objective response. Close to half of all patients in each arm had stage IV melanoma and approximately half had been previously treated. The study met its primary endpoint as the durable response rate in the T-VEC arm was significantly higher compared with the GM-CSF arm (16.3% vs 2.1%). Both the ORRs and rates of complete responders were also significantly higher in the T-VEC arm (26.4% vs 5.7% and 10.8% vs 1%, respectively). The response rate in injected metastatic lesions was 64%, whereas 34% of noninjected nonvisceral metastases and 15% of noninjected visceral metastases also responded to T-VEC. The response rates differed substantially across melanoma stages in retrospective analyses: 33% of patients with stage III melanoma had an objective response to T-VEC compared with approximately 5% of patients with stage IVM1b/c. The median overall survival showed a trend toward significance in favor of the T-VEC arm (23.3 months vs 18.9 months; hazard ratio 0.79; 95% CI, 0.62–1.00; $P = .051$). Consistent with the experience from the phase 1 and phase 2 studies, T-VEC was overall well tolerated and no new safety signals were detected. Caveats of the phase 3 study were the lack of a placebo control, the complex and (in part) subjective assessments of tumor response consisting of imaging studies, clinical assessments, and tumor biopsies as well as the choice of the comparator arm. Nevertheless, T-VEC received approval by the Food and Drug Administration for the treatment of advanced unresectable melanoma in 2015. Despite the complex logistics, including biosafety precautions and the necessity of operationalizing the tumor injections, treatment with T-VEC has been adopted widely and is offered at many academic and nonacademic institutions in the United States and elsewhere. Nevertheless, the drug remains a niche regimen that is an option only in patients who do have injectable tumors and should be considered primarily for patients with stage III or IV M1a melanoma with relatively indolent disease.

### Talimogene laherparepvec in melanoma: combination with immune checkpoint inhibitors

Given its ability to induce T-cell inflammation in metastatic tumors, T-VEC is a compelling agent to be partnered with ICI, either in earlier lines of therapy or in patients with anti–PD-1–resistant metastatic melanoma (or other cancers). Several studies combining T-VEC with either ipilimumab or pembrolizumab have already been completed, and a phase 3 trial comparing T-VEC in combination with the anti–PD-1 antibody pembrolizumab versus pembrolizumab alone (MASTERKEY-265/KEY-NOTE-034, clinicaltrials.gov NCT02263508) has completed accrual.

Combined therapy with T-VEC and ipilimumab was tested in phase 1 and phase 2 studies in patients with advanced melanoma. In the phase 1 trial, which was the first study to test oncolytic virus therapy in combination with ICI, the rates of grade 3 or higher AEs attributed to T-VEC versus ipilimumab were 15.8% and 21.1%, respectively; no new safety signals were seen; 4 of 18 patients had a CR, 5 had a PR, and 4 had stable disease (SD).[11] All responses except for one lasted for at least 6 months and responses were seen in both injected and uninjected lesions. In a randomized phase 2 study, 98 patients with advanced melanoma received T-VEC plus ipilimumab and 100 patients received ipilimumab monotherapy.[12] The ORRs in the combination arm were 39% versus 18% in the ipilimumab monotherapy arm. In patients with stage IIIb/c or stage IVM1a melanoma, the ORR were 44% in the combination versus 19% in the ipilimumab monotherapy arm. In patients with stage IVM1b or stage IVM1c melanoma, ORRs were 33% in the combination arm and 16% with ipilimumab alone; 16 of 31 (52%) patients with evaluable visceral metastases in the combination arm and 5 of 22 (23%) had decrease of visceral tumor burden. These data demonstrate that T-VEC in combination with ipilimumab had a systemic antitumor effect in visceral metastases and was effective in this more challenging subset of patients. Limitations of the study include the open-label design and the small size, resulting in small patient numbers in subgroup comparisons.

The combination of T-VEC and PD-1 inhibition is under investigation in patients with metastatic melanoma. The MASTERKEY-265 study is a phase Ib/III trial testing T-VEC in combination with pembrolizumab. In the phase Ib portion, 21 patients with advanced melanoma received 2 doses of T-VEC, followed by combined therapy with T-VEC and pembrolizumab. The treatment was well tolerated with no safety signals observed beyond toxicity expected from either of the 2 agents.[13] The most common AEs were fatigue (62%), chills (48%), and fever (43%)—these were attributed to T-VEC. Grade 3 or higher AEs attributed to pembrolizumab included grade 3 immune-related hepatitis, grade 3 aseptic meningitis, and grade 4 pneumonitis. Per investigator-assessed immune-related response criteria, the ORR was 61.9% (95% CI, 38.4%–81.9%) and the CR rate was 33.3% (95% CI, 14.6%–57.0%). More than 50% tumor regression was seen in 82% of injected lesions, 43% of noninjected non-visceral lesions, and 33% of noninjected visceral lesions; 9 of 13 patients whose baseline tumor biopsies had low $CD8^+$ T-cell infiltration or negative IFN-$\gamma$ signatures had objective responses. As discussed previously, response rates in patients with tumors lacking robust $CD8^+$ T-cell infiltration who were treated with pembrolizumab alone were low.[3] Increased $CD8^+$ T-cell infiltration in week 6 on-treatment tumor biopsies from injected lesions obtained after 2 doses of T-VEC was noted in 8 of 12 patients who responded to T-VEC plus pembrolizumab, whereas T-cell infiltrates decreased in on-treatment tumors from all 3 patients who did not respond to the combination therapy. A trend toward increased secretion of the cytotoxic T-cell marker granzyme B as assessed by immunohistochemistry as well as increased gene expression of IFN-$\gamma$ and $CD8\alpha$ was also detected in post–T-VEC and post–T-VEC plus pembrolizumab on-treatment tumor biopsies. Multiplexed immunohistochemistry analyses on serial biopsies in 13 patients showed broad changes in tumor inflammation after T-VEC. Furthermore, increased numbers of $CD4^+$ and $CD8^+$ cells in the peripheral blood were seen in a majority of patients after T-VEC. Collectively, these data demonstrate that T-VEC can induce tumor T-cell inflammation in tumors that lack a baseline T-cell infiltrate. Because both T-VEC and pembrolizumab have single-agent activity in advanced melanoma and given the small patient number, it cannot be concluded with certainty that the combination of T-VEC and pembrolizumab is synergistic. Because the lack of T-cell inflammation has been identified as a key obstacle to the efficacy PD-1 inhibition and that T-VEC seems to drive T cells into metastatic tumors, however, it is likely that the addition of T-VEC resulted in a conversion of primary resistance to response in a subset of melanoma patients receiving the combination therapy. The phase III portion of MASTERKEY-265, randomizing advanced melanoma patients to receive either pembrolizumab either alone or in combination with T-VEC, has recently completed accrual, and results are expected in the near future.

### Coxsackievirus A21 in Melanoma

Coxsackievirus A21 (CVA21) is a nongenetically modified virus that infects cells of the upper respiratory tract and causes common cold–like symptoms.[14] It has shown oncolytic properties in human cancer cell lines and xenografts of human cancers, including breast and prostate cancer.[15–17] After intratumoral injection, the virus attaches to the intracellular adhesion molecule 1 and decay acceleration factor, which are widely expressed on cancer cells, and it therefore preferentially infects cancer cells. CVA21 is under investigation as monotherapy as well as in combination with ipilimumab and pembrolizumab. In the Cocksackievirus A21 in Late Stage Melanoma (CALM) study (NCT01227551), 57 patients with treated or untreated unresectable stage IIIc–IVM1c melanoma received CVA21 intratumorally on days 1, 3, 5 and 8 and then every 3 weeks for an additional 6 injections.[18] Patients with at least 6 months' progression-free survival received up to 9 additional injections; 16 of 57 (28.1%) evaluable patients had objective responses by Immune-related Response Evaluation Criteria In Solid Tumors (irRECIST) and 21 of 57 (38.6%) patients had a progression-free survival of 6 months or longer as assessed by irRECIST. Responses in both injected and noninjected metastatic tumor lesions were observed. The regimen was overall well tolerated. In the phase 1b Melanoma Intra-Tumoral CAVATAK and Ipilimumab (MITCI) study (NCT02307149), the safety and efficacy of CVA21 combined with ipilimumab was tested in 26 patients with unresectable stage IIIb or higher melanoma.[19,20] Patients were treated with intratumoral injections of CVA21 on the same schedule as in the monotherapy study; ipilimumab was given at 3 mg/kg every 3 weeks for 4 doses beginning on day 22; 13 of the 26 patients had previously received anti–PD-1 therapy. The ORR was 38% and was higher in anti–PD-1–naïve patients. No new safety signals were observed. In the Cavatak and Pembrolizumab in Advanced Melanoma (CAPRA) trial (NCT02565992), CVA21 is being studied in combination with pembrolizumab in patients with stage IIIb or higher unresectable melanoma.[21] Patients receive CVA21 intratumorally on days 1, 3, 5, and 8 and then every 3 weeks for up to 19 injections. Pembrolizumab is given every 3 weeks at 2 mg/kg continuously. In the initial report, 8 of 11 (73%) evaluable patients had an objective response; all 5 patients with stage IVM1c disease experienced an objective response. Tumor regression was observed in both injected and noninjected metastatic sites. AEs attributed to CVA21 comprised low-grade constitutional symptoms. Although the data in both CVA21 plus ICI combination studies (MITCI and CAPRA) are only emerging, these initial reports are encouraging and have resulted in expansion of the CAPRA study to enroll up to 50 patients.

### HF10

HF10 is an attenuated herpes simplex virus 1 with a natural deletion of UL56, and the latency-associated transcript.[22,23] In a phase 1 trial assessing escalating doses of HF10 in patients with solid tumors, the drug was found well tolerated. No objective responses were observed with monotherapy; however, 3 patients with advanced melanoma had delayed responses.[24] HF10 in combination with ipilimumab was tested in 46 patients with advanced melanoma. As assessed by immune-related response criteria, 8 of 44 (18%) evaluable patients had a CR and 10 (23%) had a PR.[25]

## INTRALESIONAL THERAPY WITH TOLL-LIKE RECEPTOR 9 AGONISTS

Infectious organisms and cytolytic cells share conserved motifs called pathogen-associated molecular patterns (PAMPs). Immune cells receive activation signals through pattern recognition receptors called TLRs[26] (Fig. 2). TLR agonists are powerful immune adjuvants and have traditionally been used as a key component of cancer vaccines. Several intralesionally administered TLR9 agonists are in clinical development.

### PF-3512676 Plus Radiation in Low-grade Lymphoma

Intratumoral injection of the TLR9 agonist CpG induced systemic immunity and mediated complete regression of large disseminated lymphoma tumors in a preclinical lymphoma model.[27] In a phase 1 clinical trial (NCT00185965), 15 patients with relapsed indolent B-cell lymphoma received the CpG-enriched oligodeoxynucleotide (ODN) TLR9 agonist PF-3512676 in combination with radiotherapy.[28] PF-3512676 was injected into a solitary tumor site immediately prior to and after low-dose (4-Gy) radiation of that tumor. Intratumoral injections were then given weekly for a total of 8 doses. One CR, 3 PRs, and 2 SDs were observed and included regression of both injected and noninjected tumor sites. The treatments were well tolerated and no dose-limiting toxicities were seen. Infiltration of tumors with CD8 cells reactive to autologous tumor were observed in several of the patients.

### SD-101 in Combination with Radiation in Low-grade Lymphoma Patients

SD-101 is a synthetic class C CpG-ODN TLR9 agonist that induces strong induction of type I IFN. In a phase I/II dose escalation study, 29 patients with treatment-naïve low-grade B-cell lymphoma received intratumoral injections of SD-101 in combination with low-dose radiation (NCT02266147).[29] The primary endpoints of the study were safety

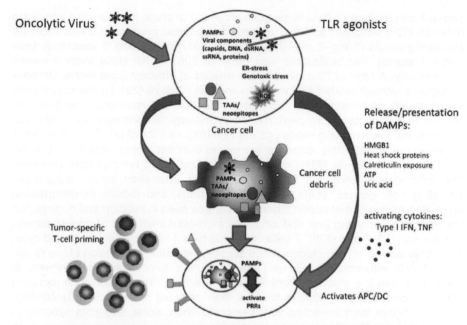

**Fig. 2.** TLR agonists (through direct stimulation of pattern recognition receptors [PRRs]) and oncolytic viral therapy (by mediating the release of PAMPs and danger-associated molecular patterns [DAMPS] with downstream stimulation of PRRs), result in activation of antigen-presenting cells and priming of tumor-specific T cells. ds, double stranded; ss, single stranded; ER, endoplasmic reticulum; ROS, reactive oxygen species; TNF, tumor necrosis factor. (*Adapted from* Woller N, Gürlevik E, Ureche CI, et al. Oncolytic viruses as anticancer vaccines. Front Oncol 2014;4:188; with permission.)

and the induction of IFN-γ–regulated genes in peripheral blood cells. Patients received low-dose radiation (4 Gy in 2 fractions given on 2 consecutive days), followed by 5 weekly injections of SD-101 into the same metastatic site. AEs were mainly comprised of flulike symptoms; 9 patients had grade 3 AEs, most of which occurred in the highest dose cohort (8 mg); 26 of the 29 evaluable patients had reduction in overall tumor burden; 7 patients had a PR and 1 patient had a CR. Regression of the radiated and injected tumor site was expected given the radiosensitivity of low-grade lymphoma; 25 of the 29 (86%) patients had regression of noninjected, nonirradiated metastatic sites; these tumor regressions, some of which deepened over time, were durable in the majority of patients. Up-regulation of IFN-γ response genes measured 24 hours after the second tumor injection was observed at all dose levels. Flow cytometry analyses of paired pretreatment and post-treatment (day 9) fine-needle aspiration samples from 16 patients with follicular lymphoma revealed increased numbers of CD3+, CD4+, and CD8+ T cells in treated lesions. Further subset analyses demonstrated a marked decrease of regulatory T cells (Tregs) and follicular T cells and a significant increase in effector CD4+ T cells. Low numbers of Tregs, and, somewhat unexpectedly, low numbers of proliferating (Ki67+) and granzyme B-positive CD8+ T cells were associated with improved clinical benefit.

## SD-101 in Combination with PD-1 Inhibition in Advanced Melanoma Patients

In a phase 1b/2 study in patients with advanced melanoma, SD-101 was tested in combination with the anti–PD-1 antibody pembrolizumab (NCT02521870).[30] In the phase 1 part, patients with unresectable stage IIIc or stage IV melanoma who were naïve to PD-1 inhibition and had at least 1 injectable metastatic lesion received escalating doses (1 mg–8 mg) of SD-101 (weekly for the first 3 injections, then every 3 weeks). Pembrolizumab was given at 200 mg flat dose every 3 weeks continuously. A total of 76 patients were treated at different dose levels. Grade 3 or higher treatment related AEs were observed in 22 of 76 (29%) patients and consisted mainly of constitutional symptoms, injection site reactions, and immune-related AEs expected from pembrolizumab therapy. Surprisingly, the ORR was higher in the lower-dose cohorts ($\leq$2 mg SD-101), with 21 of 30 (70%) of patients experiencing an objective response compared with the higher-dose cohort (8 mg SD-101), with 15 of 39 (39%) of patients responding. In retrospective analyses, this difference favoring the lower-dose cohorts was seen across subgroups, including age, gender, stage, performance status, and lactate dehydrogenase level. Regression of metastatic tumor lesions was seen in injected and noninjected visceral sites, including liver and lung. The increased infiltration of post-treatment tumors with CD4$^+$ and CD8$^+$ T cells, including type 1 helper T cells (T$_H$1) and cytotoxic cells seen in immunofluorescence studies, indicating conversion of low or absent (T-cell) inflammation into a (T-cell)–inflamed tumor microenvironment, is consistent with the mechanism of action of the drug. This observation, coupled with a response rate of 70% in the less than or equal to 2-mg SD-101 cohorts, which is higher than expected with pembrolizumab alone, suggests synergy of the combination in advanced melanoma patients.

### CMP001

CMP001 is a CpG-A ODN formulated within a virus-like particle that binds to TLR9, leading to the activation of plasmacytoid DCs.[31] In a phase 1b study (NCT02680184), patients with advanced melanoma who had either primary or acquired resistance to PD-1 inhibition were treated with intratumorally injected CMP-001 in combination with pembrolizumab. In the dose escalation phase, patients were enrolled in cohorts at 1 mg, 3 mg, 5 mg, 7.5 mg, and 10 mg of CMP-001 on 2 different schedules (weekly dosing for 7 weeks, followed by every 3 weeks' dosing or weekly for 2 weeks followed by every 3 weeks' dosing). An interim analysis of the study showed that the combined treatment was overall well tolerated; in 69 patients who were evaluable for safety, there were 9 (13%) events of hypotension and 2 (3%) events for each anemia, chills, hypotension, hypophosphatemia, and fever; 2 of 69 (3%) patients had a CR and 13 (19%) had a PR. Regression of noninjected tumors was observed in nodal, cutaneous, hepatic, and splenic metastases. Assessment of chemokines in paired baseline versus on treatment tumor biopsies was performed. A median 5.9-fold increase in CXCL10 levels over baseline was seen post-CMP001 treatment, indicating TLR9 activation. In a small subset of patients with paired pretreatment and post-treatment tumor biopsies, an increase in CD8$^+$ T-cell numbers and increased expression of PD-L1 was observed in injected and noninjected tumors. Furthermore, RNA analysis revealed up-regulation of an inflammatory gene signature preferentially in responders. These data are consistent with the mechanism of action of CMP001, demonstrating activation of plasmacytoid DCs and induction of T-cell inflammation in treated tumors.

### Tilsotolimod (IMO-2125) in Combination with Ipilimumab in Advanced Melanoma Patients

Tilsotolimod (IMO-2125) is a synthetic oligonucleotide, which targets TLR9. In the dose escalation part of the ILLUMINATE-204 study (NCT02644967), 18 patients received increasing doses of IMO-2125 (4–32 mg) in combination with ipilimumab at 3 mg/kg. In the (ongoing) phase 2 dose expansion part, patients who have progressed after PD-1 inhibition are treated with intratumoral injections of IMO-2125 at the recommended phase 2 dose of 8 mg in weeks 1, 2, 3, 5, 8, 11, 17, 23, and 29. Four doses of ipilimumab were given at weeks 2, 5, 8, and 11. In an interim report, 13 of 26 (50%) patients had at least 1 greater than or equal to grade 3 treatment-related AE. Six patients (23%) had immune-related AEs that were attributed to ipilimumab. Of the 21 patients who were assessable for response to treatment, there were 2 (9%) CRs, 6 (28.6%) PRs, and 7 (33.3%) patients with SD. Notably, 15 of the 26 patients (57.7%) had metastatic lesions that required image-guided injections. Regression was observed in injected as well as uninjected tumor lesions.

## INTRALESIONAL THERAPY WITH PROINFLAMMATORY CYTOKINES

Proinflammatory cytokines, such as IFN-$\alpha$, interleukin (IL)-2, and IL-12, have the ability to stimulate T-cell inflammation in the tumor. Systemic administration of IFN-$\alpha$ and IL-2 has had regulatory approval and has been used for many years for the treatment of melanoma and renal cell cancer; however, these agents provide clinical benefit only for a small subset of patients and are associated with substantial toxicity.[32,33] IL-12 is secreted by different immune cell subsets including DCs, macrophages, and neutrophils. In conjunction with IFN-$\gamma$, it plays a critical role in polarization of T cells toward a $T_H1$ response and during the priming and activation of T-cells against antigens, but has multiple other functions, including the survival of memory T cells, antiangiogenesis, and the inhibition of Tregs, myeloid-derived suppressor cells, and $T_H2$ responses.[34,35] Systemic IL-12 and intratumoral administration leads to $T_H1$ polarization, but has modest activity and substantial toxicity in solid tumors.[34,36]

Intratumoral (IT) Tavokinogene telseplasmid (tavo) electroporation (EP) (IT-tavo-EP) combines injection of plasmid IL-12 with subsequent electroporation, mediating localized IL-12 expression with minimal systemic exposure. Tavo encodes for both p35 and p40 subunits of the human IL-12 protein and is injected directly into the tumor. In a phase 1 study, 24 melanoma patients with unresectable, accessible lesions received 3 intratumoral injections (days 1, 5, and 8) of IT-tavo-EP.[37] Pain, erythema, and bleeding at the treatment sites were noted, but no systemic AEs attributed to IT-tavo-EP were observed. Tumor regression was seen in treated and nontreated metastatic sites; 10 of 19 patients with noninjected metastatic sites had either objective responses or SD; 2 of the objective responses were CRs. Tumor T-cell infiltration was seen in post-treatment biopsies. In a phase 2 study (OMS-I100), 51 patients with unresectable and injectable melanoma received at least 3 administrations of IT-tavo-EP into 2 to 4 tumor sites at days 1, 8, and 15. Two phase 2 studies in which IT-tavo-EP therapy is partnered with pembrolizumab are ongoing; 1 of the studies is conducted in advanced melanoma patients with noninflamed tumors (OMS-I102) and 1 in patients who have experienced progression after PD-1 inhibition (OMS-I103, NCT03132675). In the OMS-I-102 study, patients receive IT-tavo-EP on days 1, 5, and 8 of every 6-week cycle. In an interim analysis, 2 of 22 (9%) of evaluable patients had CR, 9 (41%) had PR, and 2 (9%) had SD.

## STIMULATOR OF INTERFERON GENES AGONISTS

As described in Peter Düwell and colleagues' article, "Innate Immune Stimulation In Cancer Therapy," in this issue, STING is a mitochondrial adaptor protein that is activated by the endogenous cyclic dinucleotide cGAMP on binding of cyclic guanosine monophosphate–adenosine monophosphate synthase to cytosolic DNA. Activation of

STING results in up-regulation of genes coding for type I IFNs. STING activation is a critical step in the induction of tumor-directed T-cell responses, and synthetic cyclic dinucleotides have demonstrated antitumor activity in preclinical models.[38] Several STING agonists, including ADU-S100(MIW815) and MK-1454, are currently in clinical development (NCT03172936, NCT02675439, and NCT03010176). Interim results of a phase 1 study testing MK-1454 either as monotherapy or in combination with pembrolizumab were recently reported.[39] Toxicities attributed to MK-1454 that occurred in greater than 10% of patients included, fevers, chills, pain at the injection site, fatigue, and nausea; 6 of 25 (24%) patients in the combination arm had PRs (3 patients with head and squamous cell cancer, 1 patient with triple-negative breast cancer, and 2 patients with anaplastic thyroid carcinoma). No objective responses were observed with MK-1454 monotherapy.

## PERSPECTIVE

The early clinical experience suggests that intralesional therapies have the capability to drive T cells into metastatic tumors and thus potentially convert non–T-cell inflamed tumors into T-cell inflamed ones, at least in a subset of patients. Because lack of tumor T-cell infiltration is a key barrier to the clinical efficacy of ICI (and likely other immunotherapies), and given the relatively modest single-agent activity for noninjected metastatic sites, their primary role will likely be as partnering agents with ICI and other immunotherapies. Clinical development of intralesional therapies is predominantly focused on combination therapy with ICIs. The data available to date indicate that these combinatorial approaches achieve higher response rates in ICI-naïve melanoma patients and that approximately 20% of melanoma patients with resistance to PD-1 inhibition have objective responses. Despite their distinct targets and mechanisms, the proportion of melanoma patients who achieve benefit from the addition of intratumorally injected agents seems fairly similar across studies. Given that a dominant downstream effect of intralesional therapy is the activation of an innate immune response, there may be significant overlap in the subsets of patients who can benefit from these therapies, which may be variable across different tumor types. Future biomarker-driven studies, potentially including comparisons or even combinations of different intratumoral approaches, will give more insight into mechanistic nuances and most suitable use for these therapies in cancer patients.

## REFERENCES

1. Chen DS, Mellman I. Oncology meets immunology: the cancer-immunity cycle. Immunity 2013;39(1):1–10.
2. Topalian SL, Taube JM, Anders RA, et al. Mechanism-driven biomarkers to guide immune checkpoint blockade in cancer therapy. Nat Rev Cancer 2016;16(5): 275–87.
3. Tumeh PC, Harview CL, Yearley JH, et al. PD-1 blockade induces responses by inhibiting adaptive immune resistance. Nature 2014;515(7528):568–71.
4. Cristescu R, Mogg R, Ayers M, et al. Pan-tumor genomic biomarkers for PD-1 checkpoint blockade-based immunotherapy. Science 2018;362(6411).
5. Ayers M, Lunceford J, Nebozhyn M, et al. IFN-gamma-related mRNA profile predicts clinical response to PD-1 blockade. J Clin Invest 2017;127(8):2930–40.
6. Spranger S, Gajewski TF. Impact of oncogenic pathways on evasion of antitumour immune responses. Nat Rev Cancer 2018;18(3):139–47.
7. Ott PA, Hodi FS. Talimogene laherparepvec for the treatment of advanced melanoma. Clin Cancer Res 2016;22(13):3127–31.

8. Hu JC, Coffin RS, Davis CJ, et al. A phase I study of OncoVEXGM-CSF, a second-generation oncolytic herpes simplex virus expressing granulocyte macrophage colony-stimulating factor. Clin Cancer Res 2006;12(22):6737–47.

9. Senzer NN, Kaufman HL, Amatruda T, et al. Phase II clinical trial of a granulocyte-macrophage colony-stimulating factor-encoding, second-generation oncolytic herpesvirus in patients with unresectable metastatic melanoma. J Clin Oncol 2009;27(34):5763–71.

10. Andtbacka RH, Kaufman HL, Collichio F, et al. Talimogene laherparepvec improves durable response rate in patients with advanced melanoma. J Clin Oncol 2015;33(25):2780–8.

11. Puzanov I, Milhem MM, Minor D, et al. Talimogene laherparepvec in combination with Ipilimumab in previously untreated, unresectable stage IIIB-IV melanoma. J Clin Oncol 2016;34(22):2619–26.

12. Chesney J, Puzanov I, Collichio F, et al. Randomized, open-label phase II study evaluating the efficacy and safety of talimogene laherparepvec in combination with ipilimumab versus ipilimumab alone in patients with advanced, unresectable melanoma. J Clin Oncol 2018;36(17):1658–67.

13. Ribas A, Dummer R, Puzanov I, et al. Oncolytic virotherapy promotes intratumoral T cell infiltration and improves anti-PD-1 immunotherapy. Cell 2017;170(6): 1109–19.e10.

14. Spickard A, Evans H, Knight V, et al. Acute respiratory disease in normal volunteers associated with Coxsackie A-21 viral infection. III. Response to nasopharyngeal and enteric inoculation. J Clin Invest 1963;42:840–52.

15. Shafren DR, Au GG, Nguyen T, et al. Systemic therapy of malignant human melanoma tumors by a common cold-producing enterovirus, coxsackievirus a21. Clin Cancer Res 2004;10(1 Pt 1):53–60.

16. Berry LJ, Au GG, Barry RD, et al. Potent oncolytic activity of human enteroviruses against human prostate cancer. Prostate 2008;68(6):577–87.

17. Skelding KA, Barry RD, Shafren DR. Systemic targeting of metastatic human breast tumor xenografts by Coxsackievirus A21. Breast Cancer Res Treat 2009; 113(1):21–30.

18. Andtbacka RHI, Curti BD, Kaufman H, et al. CALM study: a phase II study of an intratumorally delivered oncolytic immunotherapeutic agent, coxsackievirus A21, in patients with stage IIIc and stage IV malignant melanoma. J Clin Oncol 2014; 32:5s, suppl; abstr 3031.

19. Curti B, Richards JM, Hallmeyer S, et al. Activity of a novel immunotherapy combination of intralesional coxsackievirus A21 and systemic Ipilimumab in advanced melanoma patients previously treated with anti-PD1 blockade therapy. J Clin Oncol 2017;35:3014.

20. Curti B, Richards J, Hallmeyer S, et al. Abstract, CT114. The MITCI (Phase 1b) study: a novel immunotherapy combination of intralesional Coxsackievirus A21 and systemic ipilimumab in advanced melanoma patients with or without previous immune checkpoint therapy treatment. Ann Oncol 2017;77:CT114.

21. Silk A, Kaufman H, Gabrail N, et al. Phase 1b study of intratumoral Coxsackievirus A21 (CVA21) and systemic pembrolizumab in advanced melanoma patients: interim results of the CAPRA clinical trial. J Clin Oncol 2017. https://doi.org/10.1158/1538-7445AM2017-CT026.

22. Nishiyama Y, Kimura H, Daikoku T. Complementary lethal invasion of the central nervous system by nonneuroinvasive herpes simplex virus types 1 and 2. J Virol 1991;65(8):4520–4.

23. Eissa IR, Naoe Y, Bustos-Villalobos I, et al. Genomic signature of the natural on-colytic herpes simplex virus HF10 and its therapeutic role in preclinical and clin-ical trials. Front Oncol 2017;7:149.
24. Ferris RL, Gross ND, Nemunaitis JJ, et al. Phase I trial of intratumoral therapy using HF10, an oncolytic HSV-1, demonstrates safety in HSV+/HSV. J Clin Oncol 2014;32:6082.
25. Andtbacka RR, Ross MI, Agarwala SS, et al. Preliminary results from phase II study of combination treatment with HF10,, a replication-competent HSV-1 onco-lytic virus aliPwSI, IIIc, Or IV, melanoma UOM. Preliminary results from phase II study of combination treatment with HF10, a replication-competent HSV-1 onco-lytic virus, and ipilimumab in patients with stage IIIb, IIIc, Or IV unresectable or metastatic melanoma. J Clin Oncol 2016;34:9543.
26. Obeid J, Hu Y, Slingluff CL Jr. Vaccines, adjuvants, and dendritic cell activators–current status and future challenges. Semin Oncol 2015;42(4):549–61.
27. Varghese B, Widman A, Do J, et al. Generation of CD8+ T cell-mediated immunity against idiotype-negative lymphoma escapees. Blood 2009;114(20):4477–85.
28. Brody JD, Ai WZ, Czerwinski DK, et al. In situ vaccination with a TLR9 agonist in-duces systemic lymphoma regression: a phase I/II study. J Clin Oncol 2010; 28(28):4324–32.
29. Frank MJ, Reagan PM, Bartlett NL, et al. In situ vaccination with a TLR9 agonist and local low-dose radiation induces systemic responses in untreated indolent lymphoma. Cancer Discov 2018;8(10):1258–69.
30. Ribas AM, Hoimes C, Amin A, et al. Phase 1b/2, open label, multicenter, study of the combination of SD-101 and pembrolizumab in patients with advanced mela-noma who are naïve to anti-PD1 therapy. J Clin Oncol 2018;36(15_suppl):9513.
31. Milhem M, Gonzales R, Medina T, et al. Intratumoral toll-like receptor 9 (TLR9) agonist, CMP-001, in combination with pembrolizumab can reverse resistance to PD-1 inhibition in a phase Ib trial in subjects with advanced melanoma. 18-LB-10610-AACR CT144. 2018.
32. Kirkwood JM, Manola J, Ibrahim J, et al. A pooled analysis of eastern cooperative oncology group and intergroup trials of adjuvant high-dose interferon for mela-noma. Clin Cancer Res 2004;10(5):1670–7.
33. Schadendorf D, Vaubel J, Livingstone E, et al. Advances and perspectives in immunotherapy of melanoma. Ann Oncol 2012;23(Suppl 10):x104–8.
34. Lasek W, Zagozdzon R, Jakobisiak M. Interleukin 12: still a promising candidate for tumor immunotherapy? Cancer Immunol Immunother 2014;63(5):419–35.
35. Canton DA, Shirley S, Wright J, et al. Melanoma treatment with intratumoral elec-troporation of tavokinogene telseplasmid (pIL-12, tavokinogene telseplasmid). Immunotherapy 2017;9(16):1309–21.
36. van Herpen CM, Looman M, Zonneveld M, et al. Intratumoral administration of re-combinant human interleukin 12 in head and neck squamous cell carcinoma pa-tients elicits a T-helper 1 profile in the locoregional lymph nodes. Clin Cancer Res 2004;10(8):2626–35.
37. Daud AI, DeConti RC, Andrews S, et al. Phase I trial of interleukin-12 plasmid electro-poration in patients with metastatic melanoma. J Clin Oncol 2008;26(36):5896–903.
38. Corrales L, Glickman LH, McWhirter SM, et al. Direct activation of STING in the tumor microenvironment leads to potent and systemic tumor regression and im-munity. Cell Rep 2015;11(7):1018–30.
39. Harrington K, BJ, Ingham M, et al. Preliminary results of the first-in-human (FIH) study of MK-1454, an agonist of stimulator of interferon genes (STING), as mono-therapy or in combination with pembrolizumab. ESMO Annual Meeting. Munich, October 19-23, 2018.

# Cytokine Therapy

Ann W. Silk, MD, MS[a,b], Kim Margolin, MD[c],*

## KEYWORDS

- Cytokine • Interleukin • Interferon • Melanoma • Renal cell carcinoma

## KEY POINTS

- Cytokines mediate proliferative and activation signals in the innate and adaptive immune system and play roles in normal physiology, with tightly regulated controls of their production, localization, and activity.
- Cytokines can be exploited therapeutically but may be limited by toxicity due to the triggering of downstream molecules, including other inflammatory cytokines, and by loss of activity owing to counter-regulatory substances, including suppressive molecules that are important for normal physiologic protection from over-reaction to pathogens and cell damage as well as autoreactivity.
- The most therapeutically relevant cytokines for cancer immunotherapy seem to be the common gamma receptor (γc) cytokines, especially IL-2 and potentially IL-15, and the potent and pleiotropic IL-12.
- Cytokines are unlikely to play a major role as single agents in treatment of malignancy, but have important adjunctive functions, with great potential for therapeutic combination with other immunomodulatory strategies.

## INTRODUCTION

The complex network of cytokines controlling immune responses is an important part of regulation of the immune system (**Fig. 1**). The first step in immune cell signaling is by direct cell-to-cell contact through transmembrane proteins on both sides of the so-called immune synapse that initiate and control an intracellular signaling cascade, representing the first and second signals in the activation of a naive T cell. The third signal is provided by cytokines, molecules that further tune the immune response and control the level and duration of activation as well as modulating the impact of effector cells on target cells.

Among cytokines, interleukin-2 (IL-2) has the longest track record of clinical exploration. IL-2 produced during type 1 immune responses drives the growth, maturation, and differentiation of naive T cells into effector T cells, helper T cells, regulatory T cells

[a] Rutgers Cancer Institute of New Jersey, 195 Little Albany Street, New Brunswick, NJ 08901, USA; [b] Dana-Farber Cancer Institute, 450 Brookline Ave, Room LW503, Boston, MA 02215, USA; [c] Department of Medical Oncology, City of Hope National Medical Center, 1500 East Duarte Road, Duarte, CA 91010, USA
* Corresponding author.
E-mail address: kmargolin@coh.org

Hematol Oncol Clin N Am 33 (2019) 261–274
https://doi.org/10.1016/j.hoc.2018.12.004
0889-8588/19/© 2018 Elsevier Inc. All rights reserved.

hemonc.theclinics.com

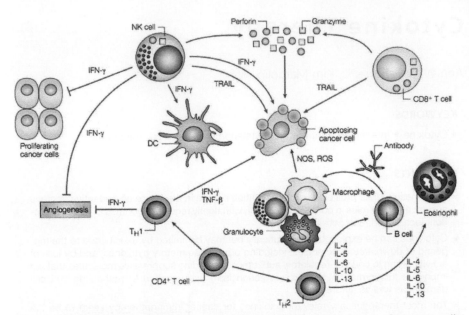

**Fig. 1.** Cytokines exert stimulatory and suppressive signals on many types of immune cells. Cytokines are usually secreted but occasionally cell bound (such as IL-15, not shown). (*From* Dranoff G. Cytokines in cancer pathogenesis and cancer therapy. Nat Rev Cancer 2004;4(1):18; with permission.)

(Tregs), and natural killer (NK) cells, which are targeted and controlled differentially by IL-2 through differences in their expression of the high ($\alpha\beta\gamma$) and intermediate ($\beta\gamma$) IL-2 receptors. NK cells and T cells become activated by $\gamma$($\gamma$c) cytokines such as IL-2, as well as by IL-12 from antigen-presenting cells (APC) to produce interferon-$\gamma$ (IFN-$\gamma$), a type II IFN, which is one of the key mediators of antitumor cytotoxicity and also a product of type 1 cells in particular. Type I IFNs, particularly IFN-$\alpha$, are critically important mediators of immune responses to virally infected cells and malignant cells. Recombinant human IFN-$\alpha$ and IL-2 are US Food and Drug Administration (FDA) approved for melanoma (adjuvant therapy) and renal cancer (advanced disease), but neither cytokine has a favorable therapeutic index owing to low single-agent activity and high frequencies of dose-related inflammatory and multi-system toxicities.

This article will focus predominantly on the cytokines with the most promise for treatment of human malignancy, including IL-2, IL-15, and IL-12. The use of IL-2 and other $\gamma$c cytokines as growth and activation factors in support of adoptive cellular therapies, such as chimeric antigen receptor-expressing T cells, will not be detailed in this article.

## TYPE 1 CYTOKINES

Cytokines are categorized as type 1, meaning they have immunostimulatory effects on T cells, and type 2, which are largely immunosuppressive. IL-2 and IFN-$\gamma$ are the prototypical type 1 cytokines, whereas IL-10 is considered to be an important type 2 cytokine. The IL-2 receptor is composed of up to 3 subunits: the IL-2R$\alpha$ (CD25), IL-2R$\beta$ (CD122), and $\gamma$c (CD132).[1] Other type 1 cytokine receptors that share $\gamma$c are IL-4, IL-7, IL-9, IL-15, IL-21, and thymic stromal lymphopoetin (**Fig. 2**). The $\gamma$c subunit is critical for normal development of the human immune system and is encoded on

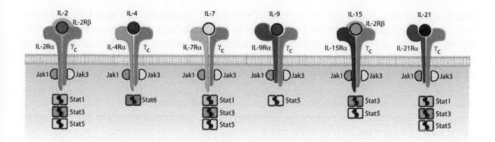

Fig. 2. Diagram of the common γ chain cytokine receptor family. The receptors for IL-2, IL-4, IL-7, IL-9, IL-15, and IL-21 share a common γ chain subunit. They transmit activation signals through JAK1/3 and various STAT proteins. (*From* Abel AM, Yang C, Thakar MS, et al. Natural killer cells: development, maturation, and clinical utilization. Front Immunol 2018;9(1869):6; with permission.)

the X chromosome. Genetic defects in the γc subunit result in X-linked severe combined immunodeficiency syndrome (SCID),[2] which is the most common form of SCID.

The receptors for IL-2 and IL-15 also share the β chain subunits, which may account for some common functions; their differences are attributed to the distribution of their cytokine-specific α receptors, which differ in their expression on different cell types and in structure and interaction with βγc. The α receptor for IL-15 is predominantly cell bound on antigen-presenting cells rather than on target cells. The IL-2α receptor confers high-affinity binding and is found preferentially on Tregs and transiently on activated lymphocytes. On resting lymphocytes, which do not express the IL-2α receptor, IL-2 binds only to intermediate-affinity βγc.

## IL-2

A recombinant human IL-2 (rhIL-2), differing by one amino acid from physiologic IL-2 (thus generically named "aldesleukin"), was FDA approved in 1992 for melanoma and in 1998 for renal cancer, based on the pooled results of phase II studies at the US National Cancer Institute (NCI) and subsequent multi-institution trials around the US. The dose and schedules were based largely on animal data showing that only very high doses given intravenously (i.v.) on cyclic schedules (giving rise to the therapeutic term high-dose IL-2 ([HD-IL-2]) could result in sufficient clinical responses, but the administration of HD-IL-2 caused severe, poorly tolerated, and reversible but often life-threatening multi-system toxicities.[3] The response rate for HD-IL-2 from pooled data in advanced melanoma patients was 16%, about half of the responses complete (most durable) and the remainder partial (some durable).[4] Based on pooled datasets, 82% of the 33 melanoma patients who had a complete response remained in continuous remission for 3+ to 11+ years of follow-up.[5] Although present-day sophisticated analyses were not possible in the era of IL-2's clinical development, IL-2-induced rebound circulating blood lymphocytosis after initial transient lymphopenia, as well as a heavy lymphocytic infiltrate into residual tumors from biopsies performed in a subset of responding patients with residual tumor,[6] supported the concept of IL-2-induced stimulation of intratumoral effector CD8 T cells as the dominant mechanism of antitumor effects. However, Tregs, which constitutively express the high-affinity αβγ receptor, are also stimulated by IL-2, even at low doses,[7] and may be a major contributor to the limited benefit of HD-IL-2.

Toxicities of HD-IL-2, reflecting its stimulation of a cascade of other inflammatory substances that include IFN-γ, tumor necrosis factor-α, IL-1, and IL-6,[8–10] can be severe and cumulative but are nearly always reversible, resolving within hours to days of stopping therapy. Most toxicities result from acute vasodilatation and hypotension, with a capillary leak syndrome that results in fluid overload and hypotension. Fever, rigors, nausea, vomiting, diarrhea, and elevation of serum creatinine and bilirubin are common. Rash and pruritus may be complicated by skin breakdown, which contributed to a high incidence of bacterial infections, particularly with *Staphylococcus aureus*, in patients treated before the routine use of antibiotics; IL-2 paradoxically leads to a suppressive effect on neutrophil chemotaxis.[11] Published IL-2 treatment guidelines provide for the clinically based selection of patients and management of IL-2 toxicities, but to date there are no satisfactory biomarkers to select patients most likely to benefit.[12]

### IL-2 in the era of checkpoint inhibition

Since the advent of the immune checkpoint-blocking CTLA-4 and PD-1 antibodies, which have a markedly superior therapeutic index over HD-IL-2, the latter is rarely if ever used as a first-line therapy and remains of uncertain benefit after failure of checkpoint blockade and, when applicable, molecularly targeted therapies (melanoma) or broadly targeted kinase inhibitors (renal cancer). However, limited data suggest that the efficacy and safety of HD-IL-2 are preserved in patients who have already received anti-CTLA4 blockade. The response rate among 52 melanoma patients who had prior ipilimumab therapy was 21%, comparable to the pooled response rates of ~16% for patients treated initially with high-dose IL-2, compared with 12% who had not received ipilimumab.[13] Toxicity in the 2 groups was roughly equivalent, which may reflect in part the selection of patients with little or no immune-related toxicity from their prior immune checkpoint blockade. HD-IL-2 has also been used as a salvage regimen following PD-1 or PD-L1 inhibition. In a cohort of melanoma patients, the response rate was 22.5% (9 of 40) and in renal cell carcinoma (RCC) patients, the response rate was 23.5% (4 of 17; unpublished data). These observations lend support to the concept of non-cross-resistance with other mechanisms and further investigations of combined therapy with IL-2 as an adjunctive agent.

### New formulations of IL-2

Patient- and tumor-based predictors of response to IL-2 therapy remain unavailable, but data in melanoma suggested a negative correlation between the presence of circulating CD4+FoxP3+ (Tregs) and response to HD-IL-2.[14] Rebound lymphocytosis is a dynamic effect of therapy that, while associated with favorable outcome, cannot be predicted at the outset. Like many cytokines, IL-2 triggers a cascade of counter-regulatory suppressive molecules that may also limit its benefits.

To address some of these limitations, novel formulations of IL-2 are in development, with promising preclinical and early clinical data. One such agent is a polyethylene glycol-modified aldesleukin that is subject in vivo to a pH-dependent controlled cleavage of all but 1 to 2 of its 6 polyethylene glycol moieties, producing an agonist that preferentially stimulates IL-2 receptor $\beta\gamma c$, resulting in stimulation of CD8 and NK cells over Tregs.[15] The safety and long half-life allows outpatient dosing every 3 weeks, an ideal regimen for combination with immune checkpoint antibodies, a strategy that is already in clinical phase III study for melanoma, and in phase II for several other malignancies, with promising early evidence of activity (NCT02983045). Other strategies include the engineering of IL-2 with a protein that targets the tumor stroma and thus preferentially stimulates intratumoral CD8 cells more than Tregs, while leaving peripheral Tregs unaffected, thus protecting the patient from immune-related toxicities, and other altered IL-2 molecules that bind only $\beta\gamma c$, with the resulting advantages detailed above for the polyethylene glycol-modified IL-2.

## IL-15

IL-15 shares the βγc receptor targeted by IL-2 and thus mediates its effect on many of the same cells and induces many similar functions. However, differences in the structure, localization, and function of their cytokine-specific α receptors account for functional distinctions, most importantly a lack of stimulation of Tregs by IL-15. IL-15 preferentially stimulates the proliferation and antitumor cytotoxic activity of NK cells (particularly the CD56-bright subset, responsible for highest production of type 1 cytokines) and memory CD8 T cells. The IL-15 α receptor (IL15RA) is generally expressed on antigen-presenting cells, predominantly dendritic cells (DC) but also neutrophils, monocytes, mast cells, B cells, and fibroblasts. The synthesis of IL15RA occurs in concert with that of IL-15 itself, which is then available in cell-bound form to ligand with the βγ receptor complex on target cells. Whereas IL-15 signaling is thus similar to that of IL-2, these differences in the distribution and interaction of α receptor chains with the βγ receptor complex control the signaling triggered by IL-2 and IL-15 and the cells most responsive to these signals. IL-15, like IL-7 (detailed below), is a "homeostatic" cytokine, playing a critical role in the control of peripheral blood lymphocyte counts by varying serum concentrations and receptor availability in response to circulating lymphocyte levels.

Preclinical studies of IL-15 have demonstrated its proliferative effects on CD8 and NK cells and its safety of administration in primate models.[16] The first studies in patients with cancer were designed to select the optimal doses, schedules, and routes of administration for further investigation. Investigators at the US NCI produced the first rhIL-15 and tested it as a single agent, demonstrating the ability of i.v. boluses given daily for 12 consecutive days to induce dynamic changes in the blood lymphocyte compartment. Immediately after rhIL-15 administration, there was a rapid efflux of NK cells and gamma delta (γδ) T cells, which are a low-frequency subset of invariant receptor-expressing effector cells with innate-like immune properties similar to NK or NK T cells. Approximately 4 hours later, an influx of these cells back into the circulation was observed, followed by proliferative expansion of NK cells (10-fold), γδ T cells (10-fold), and memory subsets of CD8 cells (3- to 10-fold), which peaked several days after the last IL-15 infusion.[17] IL-15 administered in this fashion also led to marked elevations (20- to 50-fold) of plasma IL-6 and IFN-γ concentrations. Despite the dramatic expansion of effector cell subsets in the circulation induced by IL-15, no antitumor activity was observed among 18 patients treated over a dose range of 0.3–3 µg/kg/day, and dose-limiting toxicities similar to those of IL-2—including fevers and other flu-like symptoms, hypotension, thrombocytopenia, and transaminase elevation—led to the selection of 0.3 µg/kg/day as the maximum-tolerated dose.

To further explore the potential for systemically administered rhIL-15, a follow-up study was done by investigators in the Cancer Immunotherapy Trials Network using daily subcutaneous (s.c.) administration of rhIL-15 for 5 consecutive days followed by 2 days of rest and then another 5 days of therapy.[18] Nineteen patients with a variety of adult malignancies were treated in a classic phase I dose-escalation design. As expected, the s.c. route was much better tolerated than the i.v. route, and the maximum-tolerated dose (MTD) was determined to be 2 µg/kg/day, which is 6-fold higher than with i.v. administration. In response to this route and schedule of IL-15, there was a 13.5-fold increase in circulating NK cells and a 2.8-fold increase in CD8+ T cells with a memory phenotype. Again, no objective antitumor responses were observed, although one patient with previously progressive renal cell cancer remained on therapy for 2 years with stable disease. Although the design of phase I immunotherapy studies has subsequently moved away from testing new agents as late-line therapies, which almost never show activity even for agents with activity in earlier-line therapy, sufficient data on the mechanisms and limitations of unmodified rhIL-15 emerged during these studies to quench enthusiasm about its further development as a single agent, so ongoing and future combination studies are based more directly on informative animal models.

To create an improved IL-15 agent that would retain its normal physiology with enhanced pharmacologic properties, a "superagonist" mutant form of IL-15 with an asparagine to aspartic acid substitution at amino acid 72 (N72D), which has a 4- to 5-fold increase in biologic activity, was engineered into a cytokine receptor complex containing 2 molecules of the IL-15 mutein fused to 2 molecules of the "sushi" domain of IL15RA and the Fc receptor domain of a single immunoglobulin G1 (IgG1) molecule.[19] In animal studies, this complex, also known as ALT-803, has a markedly increased half-life of 25 hours when administered i.v. compared with the 40-minute half-life of unmodified rhIL-15. After demonstrating the favorable pharmacologic and immunologic properties, as well as substantial improvements in antitumor activity of this fusion complex over rhIL-15 in several animal models, the complex entered studies in adult solid tumor patients and a group of adults with hematologic malignancies in relapse after allogeneic hematopoietic cell transplant free of active graft-versus-host disease. ALT-803 was initially administered i.v. (from 0.3 to 6 μg/kg) and then subcutaneously (from 6 to 20 μg/kg) on a weekly schedule and demonstrated a favorable safety profile, although, like the unmodified NCI rhIL-15, patients treated at the highest i.v. doses did experience inflammatory and hemodynamic effects similar to those resulting from treatment with IL-2.[20] The half-life of i.v. ALT-803 was less than 4 hours, without accumulation or loss with repeated dosing cycles. Subcutaneous administration of ALT-803 achieved a peak concentration that was 100 times lower than that of i.v. administration. Drug levels peaked 4–8 hours after s.c. administration in 4 of 8 patients, and, in the other 4 patients, the drug level was still increasing 24 hours after s.c. administration. The half-life is not known because blood was not collected beyond 24 hours, but it was markedly longer compared with i.v. dosing. The s.c. route was chosen for further study, which is now focused on combinations that exploit the expansion of NK (2- to 8-fold) and CD8 T cells (3- to 6-fold) resulting from well-tolerated s.c. dosing of ALT-803, which caused only a brisk and broad local inflammatory reaction around the sites of injection. Again, when given to patients with one of several solid tumor types who had been extensively pretreated, no objective responses were observed. Nevertheless, ALT-803 is now in trials with monoclonal antibodies for B cell malignancies, with bacillus Calmette–Guérin intravesically for recurrent non-muscle-invasive bladder cancer (NCT02138734, NCT03022825), and with immune checkpoint antibodies in selected other malignancies, using the recommended phase II/combination dose of 20 μg/kg given weekly for 4–5 weeks. Some of these pilot studies have been published: ALT-803 plus the PD-1 antibody nivolumab was administered to 21 patients with non-small-cell lung cancer and showed activity in checkpoint antibody-naive patients as well as in patients not benefiting from immune checkpoint blockade. Initial immunologic studies demonstrated the anticipated expansion of NK cells without Treg expansion.[21]

## IL-12

IL-12 is a pro-inflammatory heterodimeric cytokine mainly secreted by antigen-presenting cells in response to pathogen-associated molecular patterns. IL-12 increases IFN-γ production by NK cells and promotes the polarization of immune effector cell responses toward a type 1, antitumor pattern (**Fig. 3**).[22] IL-12 is thus considered a "bridging" cytokine, mediating communications triggered by

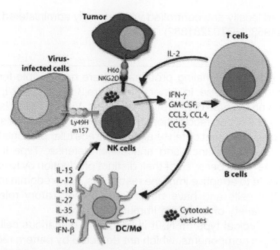

**Fig. 3.** IL-15 and IL-12 promote NK cells. NK cells receive multiple inputs, including IL-15 and IL-12, from multiple sources and, in response, make more cytokines and mediate cytotoxicity. (*From* Abel AM, Yang C, Thakar MS, et al. Natural killer cells: development, maturation, and clinical utilization. Front Immunol 2018;9(1869):8; with permission.)

inflammation-promoting substances (so-called "danger" signals required for the development of optimal adaptive, or antigen-specific/memory-capable immune responses). At the time of its initial development, before the era of immune checkpoint blockade, rhIL-12 seemed to be a promising anticancer cytokine in numerous animal models,[23] including combinations with cytotoxic chemotherapy.[24]

The first human studies of systemic rhIL-12, performed in the era following the modest success of HD-IL-2, used an initial safety-testing/pharmacokinetics-enabling i.v. dose, followed 2 weeks later by dosing once daily for 5 days every 3 weeks to establish the MTD in patients with advanced melanoma or renal cancer.[25] Subsequently, the initial dose and washout period were omitted, and unexpected systemic inflammatory toxicities occurred at doses that had been well tolerated in patients receiving the initial dose, including 2 deaths from cardiovascular collapse.[26] An analysis of serum cytokines in each group demonstrated that IL-12 induces a potent counter-regulatory cytokine reaction mediated by IL-10 (a type 2 cytokine), and the test dose had been sufficient to blunt the toxicities of subsequent IL-12 doses, a protective effect that did not occur in the phase 2 studies. The development of IL-12 as a systemic therapy was halted in favor of investigating alternative routes of administration, particularly intratumoral injection that might produce a potent local antigen-specific immune response that could lead to the development of systemic immunity and thus result in distant tumor regressions. The most promising product, with modest single-agent activity in injected lesions and occasional regression of uninjected lesions, consists of a plasmid engineered to express the IL-12 gene that is injected intratumorally and followed with local electroporation, which enhances tumor cell uptake and expression of the plasmid gene.[27] With the advent of highly active immune checkpoint-blocking antibodies in the last decade, and further studies showing the limited activity of any single-agent cytokine, combinations of checkpoint blockade with various immunomodulatory cytokines, such as this form of IL-12, have been initiated (NCT03132675). Additional formulations of IL-12 designed to limit systemic toxicity include an immunocytokine made by fusing 2 IL-12 molecules to an IgG1 antibody against tumor necrosis factor (NHS-IL12) and an adenovirus-expressing IL-12 that can be injected locally and controlled with an orally administered activator ligand switch (NCT02994953, NCT03281382).

## IFNα and IFNγ

Interferons are a group of signaling proteins that are responsible for regulating and activating the immune response. In general, there are 3 types, types I, II, and III, which are grouped based on the type of receptors they bind. Virtually all cells in the body can express type I and III IFNs on recognition of viral components, such as naked DNA or RNA, and IFNs are an important defense against intracellular pathogens. They are also important in immune surveillance and anticancer defense. Type II IFNs, originally designated "immune" IFNs because of their distinct production by lymphocytes during the bridge from innate to adaptive immune responses, are predominantly produced by NK, CD4, and CD8 cells and have major immunomodulatory roles that are also exploited in a wide variety of assays in immune-oncology.

IFN-α is the prototypical type I IFN. It is produced by various cells in the body in response to pathogen components, which are detected by pattern recognition receptors, such as Toll-like receptors. IFN-α interferes with viral replication by promoting apoptosis in the infected cell, and it also activates macrophages and NK cells. IFN-α has been used to treat a variety of malignancies over the years, including indolent B cell lymphoma and hairy-cell leukemia, chronic myelogenous leukemia (CML), RCC, and melanoma. In advanced RCC it was approved for use with bevacizumab,[28] but its contribution to the effect of the combined regimen was never well studied; its use was limited and quickly eclipsed by the arrival of anti-angiogenic tyrosine kinase inhibitors for RCC. In melanoma, IFN-α was used for more than a decade in the adjuvant setting, consistently demonstrating a modest delay in recurrence of disease with minimal impact on overall survival.[29] In melanoma, the use of IFN-α has been practically abandoned with the remarkable activity and tolerance of immune checkpoint antibodies for adjuvant treatment of high-risk resected melanoma.[30,31] A pegylated form with a long half-life suitable for s.c. dosing has also been approved and used extensively for viral hepatitis and CML, but both diseases are now more safely, tolerably, and effectively treated with small-molecule oral agents.

IFN-γ is the prototypical type II IFN. IFN-γ binds to its cell surface receptor IFNGR1/2, which is expressed on all nucleated cells and signals through the JAK-STAT1 pathway. Following activation of the receptor, STAT1 binds to the DNA at the IFN-γ activation site (GAS) and results in transcription of a cache of genes called IFN-stimulated genes. These gene products mediate the key IFN-γ functions of defense against intracellular pathogens and tumor immunosurveillance, polarization of macrophages to the M1 phenotype, and increased antigen presentation in the context of major histocompatibility complex class I. IFN-γ also has direct antitumor effects when produced locally by immune effector cells, and mutational loss of its signaling molecules in tumor cells was recently demonstrated to be an important mechanism of resistance to treatment with checkpoint inhibitors. IFN-γ mediates the increased expression of PD-L1 on tumor and other cells of the immune tumor microenvironment, and intratumoral IFN-γ production is a key predictor of response to immune checkpoint blockade[32] as well as an on-treatment marker of immune activation. Sustained IFN-γ release is associated with auto-immune conditions and macrophage activation syndrome (MAS), characterized by symptoms including fever, hepatosplenomegaly, lymphadenopathy, pancytopenia, and liver dysfunction. Systemic, unmodified IFN-γ is not suitable for therapeutic use in patients with cancer owing to a multitude of off-target side effects, such as those seen in MAS, and because IFN-γ, like IL-12, can also induce a strong counter-regulatory type 2 response.

## IL-7

IL-7 is another common γ chain receptor cytokine with a cytokine-specific α receptor heterodimerically associated with the γc receptor, which is a growth factor for naive and memory T cells. IL-7, produced predominantly by thymic epithelial cells but also by lymph node stromal cells, increases T cell receptor (TCR) diversity and promotes antigen-specific vaccine responses without stimulating Tregs.[33] IL-7 and IL-15 are denoted the "homeostatic cytokines" that regulate lymphocyte production and survival and promote the conversion from effector into memory cells.[34] When the lymphocyte count drops, as with lymphodepleting chemotherapy, IL-7 and IL-15 levels increase in a reciprocal fashion.[35] Mice with an IL-7 gene knockout develop an SCID phenotype,[36] and, in humans, an autosomal recessive form of SCID has been attributed to mutational loss of IL-7 α receptors that limit thymopoiesis. In this form of SCID, T cells are absent, but B cells and NK cells are found in normal numbers, reflecting the fact that IL-7 is important for T cell development but has minimal to no direct impact on B cells or NK cells.

Given its role in promoting memory T cells, IL-7 was tested for its potential antitumor activity. Sixteen adult patients with refractory solid tumors received rhIL-7 subcutaneously every other day for 2 weeks in a phase I dose-escalation study.[37,38] Treatment with IL-7 was associated with an excellent safety profile across doses ranging from 3 to 60 μg/kg/dose. The most common side effects were mild to moderate constitutional symptoms and mild local reactions with erythema, pruritus, and skin induration. Radiographic evidence of splenomegaly and lymphadenopathy were observed, consistent with the lymphoproliferative effect of IL-7, which was reversible. IL-7 treatment also resulted in a 2- to 4-fold increase in peripheral CD4+ and CD8+ lymphocytes at the 2 highest doses. TCR diversity spectratype analysis in 6 patients at the higher doses demonstrated that the TCR on CD4+, CD8+, or both types of lymphocytes, became significantly more diverse in 4 of the 6 patients, suggesting that naive T cells were expanded and matured after rhIL-7 treatment. Although no clinical antitumor responses were seen in the dose-escalation study, the ability of IL-7 to broaden the TCR repertoire and support T cell memory and antigen-specific responses has kept interest high, and IL-7 is currently under investigation as an adjunct to dendritic cell vaccine-based strategies (NCT01881867), checkpoint blockade (NCT03513952), and chemoradiotherapy (NCT02659800). IL-7 is also of particular interest in HIV-associated malignancies, in which the promotion of lymphopoiesis and the development of memory and a broadened TCR repertoire may be particularly important in the control of malignancy.

## IL-10

IL-10 is produced by T cells and dendritic cells. It is a pleiotropic cytokine that inhibits the secretion of pro-inflammatory cytokines at lower concentrations; but, at higher concentrations, it activates CD8+ cells in the tumor microenvironment and induces their proliferation. IL-10 also acts on CD4+ cells, Tregs, NK cells, and dendritic cells. In several mouse models, i.v. treatment with an IL-10-containing plasmid induced expansion of tumor-resident CD8+ T cells and induced tumor rejection.[39] The frequency of CD8+ TILs producing IFN-γ increased 3-fold on IL-10 treatment. Blockade of T cell trafficking from lymphoid organs into the tumor did not impair the IL-10-induced CD8+ T cell response, suggesting that the effect of IL-10 is specific to the preexisting intratumoral T cells.

IL-10 has a short half-life. To improve the pharmacokinetic and pharmacodynamic properties for use as a cancer immunotherapy, a pegylated form was developed.

Pegylation enables higher sustained serum concentrations and seems to retain the same immunologic effects. The pegylated form, pegilodecakin (PEGylated hIL-10, AM0010), was evaluated for its safety and activity in patients in a phase I study. In the dose-expansion cohort of heavily pretreated RCC patients 4 of 15 (27%) evaluable patients achieved a partial response following treatment with i.v. AM0010 at a dose of 20 µg/kg daily (s.c. injection).[40] Analysis of patient blood samples showed expansion of novel T cell clones, which correlated with objective tumor response.[41] Proliferation and expansion of LAG-3+ PD-1+ T cells also correlated with objective tumor response, suggesting a role for checkpoint antibodies in combination with pegylated IL-10.

## GM-CSF

Granulocyte macrophage colony-stimulating factor (GM-CSF) recruits and activates antigen-presenting cells, which process and present tumor-derived antigens to promote an effector T cell response. Talimogene laherparepvec (T-VEC) is an attenuated herpes simplex virus type 1 (HSV-1) carrying the gene for human GM-CSF.[42] The intratumoral administration of this engineered HSV leads to tumor cell production of high levels of GM-CSF locally, which attracts antigen-presenting cells by chemotaxis and leads to a local adaptive immune response to tumor antigens that can also produce tumor control distant from the site of injection. In animal models, this strategy also conferred protection against rechallenge with the same tumor.[43] The agent was recently approved by the US FDA for advanced melanoma amenable to intratumoral injection, based on the data from a phase III study in which 436 patients were randomly assigned to receive intratumoral T-VEC or s.c. recombinant GM-CSF as a comparator.[42] All patients were required to have measurable distant disease as well as an injectable tumor. The durable (>6 months) *overall* response rate (including lesional plus distant metastases) was significantly higher in the T-VEC arm compared with the s.c. GM-CSF arm (16.3% vs 2.1%, P<.001), and there was a borderline improvement of overall survival for T-VEC.[42] Although the response rate in injected lesions was excellent, responses were relatively infrequent in distant disease, particularly in visceral organ metastases.[44]

Subsequent trials have been designed to test the value of adding intratumoral T-VEC to immune checkpoint blockade. Initial data in melanoma are encouraging, with a randomized phase II study of 198 advanced melanoma patients treated with T-VEC and ipilimumab showing a response rate of 39% compared with 18% with ipilimumab alone.[45] In a phase Ib pilot study of T-VEC and systemic pembrolizumab in 21 anti-PD-1 naive patients, responses were seen in 62% of patients. A phase III study of T-VEC with pembrolizumab has been fully accrued but not yet analyzed. Many similar trials of other novel intralesional therapies in melanoma and other malignancies have been designed to test the value of local intratumoral therapy to prevent or reverse resistance to systemic immunotherapy. Cytokines that are used systemically and detailed earlier in this article have also been used intralesionally, including IL-2 and both type 1 (α and β) and type 2 (γ) IFNs, but the data for their activity and dose/route-related toxicities are mainly anecdotal and of uncertain broad applicability.

## SUMMARY

Cytokines are powerful and critical mediators of normal immune system function. The therapeutic use of recombinant human cytokines represented a proof of principle to the field of cancer immunotherapy and a modestly successful anticancer strategy for many years, particularly with HD-IL-2, which was considered from the 1990s until approximately 2010 to be the only FDA-approved therapy with curative potential for advanced melanoma and renal cell cancer. Even the studies of the earliest form of adoptive cell therapy for solid tumors, autologous tumor-infiltrating lymphocytes, required lymphodepleting chemotherapy and brief exposure to HD-IL-2 (as well as IL-2 in the preparative cultures) to maximize the persistence and activity of the therapeutic cell product following infusion; and the lymphodepletion is believed to work predominantly by triggering the production of the homeostatic $\gamma c$ cytokines IL-7 and IL-15. Despite the power and promise of cytokine therapy in human cancer, systemic delivery is not effective for most treated patients and is often limited by substantial toxicity. Unmodified cytokines such as IL-2 and IFN-$\gamma$ are powerful but blunt tools. Multiple new approaches seek to refine both the efficacy and the toxicity of cytokines for treatment of malignancy. New cytokine constructs are being engineered by fusing them with receptor proteins to increase their specificity or enhance pharmacodynamic and pharmacokinetic properties compared with the parent cytokine, such as the IL-15 superagonist ALT-803 (renamed N-803). Another approach is to incorporate native-form or engineered cytokines as an adjunct to complementary immunotherapy approaches such as immune checkpoint blockade, oncolytic viral therapy, adoptive T cell therapy, and tumor vaccines. Novel delivery platforms such as in an oncolytic virus (eg, T-VEC), or an intratumoral electroporation, as in the case of IL-12, may hold promise for further definition of the optimal strategies and their best application in selected malignancies and settings (such as neo-adjuvant approaches and adjuvant therapies, which have been little investigated for these agents). Future studies for cancer immunotherapy will be best served by moving away from the systemic administration of native-form cytokines, as well as by investigating the complex mechanisms of their action and surmountable challenges to their application in human malignant disease.

## REFERENCES

1. Liao W, Lin J-X, Leonard Warren J. Interleukin-2 at the crossroads of effector responses, tolerance, and immunotherapy. Immunity 2013;38(1):13–25.
2. Noguchi M, Yi H, Rosenblatt HM, et al. Interleukin-2 receptor $\gamma$ chain mutation results in X-linked severe combined immunodeficiency in humans. Cell 1993;73(1):147–57.
3. Rosenberg SA, Lotze MT, Muul LM, et al. Observations on the systemic administration of autologous lymphokine-activated killer cells and recombinant interleukin-2 to patients with metastatic cancer. N Engl J Med 1985;313(23):1485–92.
4. Atkins M, Lotze M, Dutcher J, et al. High dose recombinant interleukin 2 therapy for patients with metastatic melanoma: analysis of 270 patients treated between 1985 and 1993. J Clin Oncol 1999;17:2105–16.
5. Rosenberg SA, Yang JC, White DE, et al. Durability of complete responses in patients with metastatic cancer treated with high-dose interleukin-2: identification of the antigens mediating response. Ann Surg 1998;228(3):307–19.
6. Lotze MT, Chang AE, Seipp CA, et al. High-dose recombinant interleukin 2 in the treatment of patients with disseminated cancer. Responses, treatment-related morbidity, and histologic findings. JAMA 1986;256(22):3117–24.
7. Yu A, Zhu L, Altman N, et al. A low interleukin-2 receptor signaling threshold supports the development and homeostasis of T regulatory cells. Immunity 2009;30(2):204–17.
8. Economou JS, Hoban M, Lee JD, et al. Production of tumor necrosis factor alpha and interferon gamma in interleukin-2-treated melanoma patients: correlation with clinical toxicity. Cancer Immunol Immunother 1991;34(1):49–52.

9. Siegel JP, Puri RK. Interleukin-2 toxicity. J Clin Oncol 1991;9(4):694–704.
10. Weidmann E, Bergmann L, Stock J, et al. Rapid cytokine release in cancer patients treated with interleukin-2. J Immunother 1992;12(2):123–31.
11. Kammula US, White DE, Rosenberg SA. Trends in the safety of high dose bolus interleukin-2 administration in patients with metastatic cancer. Cancer 1998;83(4):797–805.
12. Dutcher JP, Schwartzentruber DJ, Kaufman HL, et al. High dose interleukin-2 (Aldesleukin) - expert consensus on best management practices - 2014. J Immunother Cancer 2014;2(1):26.
13. Buchbinder EI, Gunturi A, Perritt J, et al. A retrospective analysis of high-dose interleukin-2 (HD IL-2) following ipilimumab in metastatic melanoma. J Immunother Cancer 2016;4:52.
14. Cesana GC, DeRaffele G, Cohen S, et al. Characterization of CD4$^+$CD25$^+$ regulatory T cells in patients treated with high-dose interleukin-2 for metastatic melanoma or renal cell carcinoma. J Clin Oncol 2006;24(7):1169–77.
15. Charych DH, Hoch U, Langowski JL, et al. NKTR-214, an engineered cytokine with biased IL2 receptor binding, increased tumor exposure, and marked efficacy in mouse tumor models. Clin Cancer Res 2016;22(3):680–90.
16. Waldmann TA, Lugli E, Roederer M, et al. Safety (toxicity), pharmacokinetics, immunogenicity, and impact on elements of the normal immune system of recombinant human IL-15 in rhesus macaques. Blood 2011;117(18):4787–95.
17. Conlon KC, Lugli E, Welles HC, et al. Redistribution, hyperproliferation, activation of natural killer cells and CD8 T cells, and cytokine production during first-in-human clinical trial of recombinant human interleukin-15 in patients with cancer. J Clin Oncol 2015;33(1):74–82.
18. Miller JS, Morishima C, McNeel DG, et al. A first-in-human phase 1 study of subcutaneous outpatient recombinant human IL-15 (rhIL-15) in adults with advanced solid tumors. Clin Cancer Res 2018;24(7):1525–35.
19. Han K-P, Zhu X, Liu B, et al. IL-15:IL-15 receptor alpha superagonist complex: high-level co-expression in recombinant mammalian cells, purification and characterization. Cytokine 2011;56(3):804–10.
20. Margolin K, Morishima C, Velcheti V, et al. Phase I trial of ALT-803, a novel recombinant IL15 complex, in patients with advanced solid tumors. Clin Cancer Res 2018;24(22):5552–61.
21. Wrangle JM, Velcheti V, Patel MR, et al. ALT-803, an IL-15 superagonist, in combination with nivolumab in patients with metastatic non-small cell lung cancer: a non-randomised, open-label, phase 1b trial. Lancet Oncol 2018;19(5):694–704.
22. Vignali DAA, Kuchroo VK. IL-12 family cytokines: immunological playmakers. Nat Immunol 2012;13:722.
23. Brunda MJ, Luistro L, Warrier RR, et al. Antitumor and antimetastatic activity of interleukin 12 against murine tumors. J Exp Med 1993;178(4):1223–30.
24. Nars MS, Kaneno R. Immunomodulatory effects of low dose chemotherapy and perspectives of its combination with immunotherapy. Int J Cancer 2013;132(11):2471–8.
25. Atkins MB, Robertson MJ, Gordon M, et al. Phase I evaluation of intravenous recombinant human interleukin 12 in patients with advanced malignancies. Clin Cancer Res 1997;3(3):409–17.
26. Leonard JP, Sherman ML, Fisher GL, et al. Effects of single-dose interleukin-12 exposure on interleukin-12-associated toxicity and interferon-γ production. Blood 1997;90(7):2541–8.

27. Daud AI, DeConti RC, Andrews S, et al. Phase I trial of interleukin-12 plasmid electroporation in patients with metastatic melanoma. J Clin Oncol 2008;26(36): 5896–903.

28. Escudier B, Bellmunt J, Négrier S, et al. Phase III trial of bevacizumab plus interferon alfa-2a in patients with metastatic renal cell carcinoma (AVOREN): final analysis of overall survival. J Clin Oncol 2010;28(13):2144–50.

29. Eggermont AMM, Suciu S, Santinami M, et al. Adjuvant therapy with pegylated interferon alfa-2b versus observation alone in resected stage III melanoma: final results of EORTC 18991, a randomised phase III trial. Lancet 2008;372(9633): 117–26.

30. Eggermont AMM, Chiarion-Sileni V, Grob J-J, et al. Prolonged survival in stage III melanoma with ipilimumab adjuvant therapy. N Engl J Med 2016;375(19): 1845–55.

31. Eggermont AMM, Blank CU, Mandala M, et al. Adjuvant pembrolizumab versus placebo in resected stage III melanoma. N Engl J Med 2018;378(19):1789–801.

32. Cristescu R, Mogg R, Ayers M, et al. Pan-tumor genomic biomarkers for PD-1 checkpoint blockade-based immunotherapy. Science 2018;362(6411) [pii: eaar3593].

33. Lévy Y, Sereti I, Tambussi G, et al. Effects of recombinant human interleukin 7 on T-cell recovery and thymic output in HIV-infected patients receiving antiretroviral therapy: results of a phase I/IIa randomized, placebo-controlled, multicenter study. Clin Infect Dis 2012;55(2):291–300.

34. Kaech SM, Tan JT, Wherry EJ, et al. Selective expression of the interleukin 7 receptor identifies effector CD8 T cells that give rise to long-lived memory cells. Nat Immunol 2003;4:1191.

35. Gattinoni L, Finkelstein SE, Klebanoff CA, et al. Removal of homeostatic cytokine sinks by lymphodepletion enhances the efficacy of adoptively transferred tumor-specific CD8+ T cells. J Exp Med 2005;202(7):907–12.

36. von Freeden-Jeffry U, Vieira P, Lucian LA, et al. Lymphopenia in interleukin (IL)-7 gene-deleted mice identifies IL-7 as a nonredundant cytokine. J Exp Med 1995; 181(4):1519–26.

37. Sportès C, Hakim FT, Memon SA, et al. Administration of rhIL-7 in humans increases in vivo TCR repertoire diversity by preferential expansion of naive T cell subsets. J Exp Med 2008;205(7):1701–14.

38. Sportès C, Babb RR, Krumlauf MC, et al. Phase I study of recombinant human interleukin-7 administration in subjects with refractory malignancy. Clin Cancer Res 2010;16(2):727–35.

39. Emmerich J, Mumm JB, Chan IH, et al. IL-10 directly activates and expands tumor-resident CD8(+) T cells without de novo infiltration from secondary lymphoid organs. Cancer Res 2012;72(14):3570–81.

40. Naing A, Papadopoulos KP, Autio KA, et al. Safety, antitumor activity, and immune activation of pegylated recombinant human interleukin-10 (AM0010) in patients with advanced solid tumors. J Clin Oncol 2016;34(29):3562–9.

41. Naing A, Infante JR, Papadopoulos KP, et al. PEGylated IL-10 (Pegilodecakin) induces systemic immune activation, CD8(+) T cell invigoration and polyclonal T cell expansion in cancer patients. Cancer Cell 2018;34(5):775–91.e3.

42. Andtbacka RHI, Kaufman HL, Collichio F, et al. Talimogene laherparepvec improves durable response rate in patients with advanced melanoma. J Clin Oncol 2015;33(25):2780–8.

43. Liu BL, Robinson M, Han ZQ, et al. ICP34.5 deleted herpes simplex virus with enhanced oncolytic, immune stimulating, and anti-tumour properties. Gene Ther 2003;10:292.
44. Kaufman HL, Amatruda T, Reid T, et al. Systemic versus local responses in melanoma patients treated with talimogene laherparepvec from a multi-institutional phase II study. J Immunother Cancer 2016;4:12.
45. Chesney J, Puzanov I, Collichio F, et al. Randomized, open-label phase II study evaluating the efficacy and safety of talimogene laherparepvec in combination with ipilimumab versus ipilimumab alone in patients with advanced, unresectable melanoma. J Clin Oncol 2018;36(17):1658–67.

# Immunotherapy Toxicity

Charlene M. Mantia, MD[a], Elizabeth I. Buchbinder, MD[b],*

## KEYWORDS

- Immunotherapy • Toxicity • Immune checkpoint inhibitors
- Immune-related adverse events

## KEY POINTS

- Advances in immunotherapy have improved treatment for patients with many types of malignancy.
- Immune checkpoint inhibitors are associated with unique side effects that can involve almost any organ system.
- Immune-related adverse events can limit further treatment options and can cause significant morbidity and mortality.

## INTRODUCTION

Recent scientific advancements have led to substantial progress in the understanding of the immune system's ability to control cancer. With these advancements, novel therapies have been developed that manipulate the immune response against cancer. These approaches include innovative vaccines, modified immune cells, antibodies, and drugs that target immune cell signaling. In particular, immune checkpoint inhibitors (ICIs) have demonstrated activity in many malignancies and are currently approved for many cancer indications.

ICIs target T-cell interactions with antigen-presenting cells (APCs) through cytotoxic T-lymphocyte associated protein-4 (CTLA-4) or through T-cell interactions with normal tissue cells, APCs, and tumor cells through programmed death-1 (PD-1) or programmed death ligand-1 (PD-L1). Ipilimumab, which targets CTLA-4, was the first ICI that was approved by the Food and Drug Administration based on improved overall survival in metastatic melanoma patients in phase 3 trials.[1] Nivolumab and pembrolizumab, which target PD-1, have demonstrated benefit in melanoma, non–small cell

Disclosure Statement: C.M. Mantia has nothing to disclose; E.I. Buchbinder receives clinical trial support from BMS, Merck, Novartis, Lilly, and Checkmate and consulting payments from BMS, Checkmate.
[a] Division of Hematology and Oncology, Beth Israel Deaconess Medical Center, Harvard Medical School, 330 Brookline Avenue, Boston, MA 02215, USA; [b] Department of Medical Oncology, Dana-Farber Cancer Institute, Harvard Medical School, Dana 2, 450 Brookline Avenue, Boston, MA 02215, USA
* Corresponding author.
E-mail address: Elizabeth_Buchbinder@DFCI.HARVARD.EDU

lung cancer, renal cell carcinoma, classical Hodgkin lymphoma, squamous cell carcinoma of the head and neck, urothelial carcinoma, advanced gastric cancer, microsatellite instable or mismatch repair–deficient solid tumors, and hepatocellular carcinoma.[2–5] Atezolizumab, avelumab, and durvalumab, which target PD-L1, have been approved for use in bladder cancer, gastric cancer, Merkel cell cancer, and platinum-resistant urothelial carcinoma.[6] In addition, combination CTLA-4 blockade and PD-1 blockade are approved in the treatment of metastatic melanoma and renal cell carcinoma.[7]

The toxicity profile of ICI differs greatly from those observed with traditional chemotherapy or targeted therapy. Immune-related adverse events can require prolonged treatment with immunosuppression, which carries its own health risks and associated morbidity. Some of the immune reactions can lead to permanent organ damage or even death. These side effects frequently lead to treatment discontinuation and may limit subsequent treatment options.

## THE PATHOPHYSIOLOGY OF IMMUNE CHECKPOINT INHIBITORS– RELATED TOXICITY

To function effectively, the immune system must be able to recognize self from nonself; there are several mechanisms that protect the host from developing autoimmune conditions. T cells that recognize the body's own proteins as foreign are deleted through negative selection in the thymus, a process termed central tolerance.[8] In the peripheral blood, spleen, and lymphatic organs T cells are exposed to professional APCs that may display self or foreign antigens. Peripheral tolerance mechanisms prevent T cells that recognize self-proteins from inflicting damage to self-tissues.[8,9]

ICIs act upon CTLA-4, PD-1, or other inhibitory pathways affecting peripheral immune tolerance. Notably, autoimmune toxicities can be induced by immunotherapies other than ICIs and can be triggered through various mechanisms. Antibody therapy may lead to innate immune damage due to complement activation or macrophage activity through antibody-dependent cell-mediated cytotoxicity. In patients treated with adoptive cell therapy, T cells may recognize antigens that are expressed on normal and tumor tissues. Immunotherapy may lead to the dysregulation of immune hemostasis by increasing immune cells not associated with the antitumor response that then attacks normal tissue. Cancer vaccines and immune adjuvants can lead to epitope spreading, thereby inducing a reaction against normal tissue.[10]

It has been postulated that immune-related adverse events are associated with antitumor response. Early studies suggested an association, but further analysis has been mixed to date.[11] One of the few side effects whereby numerous studies support an association with response is vitiligo in the case of melanoma.[12–14]

Immune-related toxicities often develop well after treatment initiation, following patterns that vary greatly from other cancer therapies.[15] The type, incidence, and severity of immune-related adverse events differ between CTLA-4 and PD-1/PD-L1 inhibitors.[15,16] Although there is minimal, if any, relation between dose and toxicity with PD-1/PD-L1 inhibition, the incidence and severity of immune-related adverse events have been shown to be dose related for the anti- CTLA-4 antibody ipilimumab.[17]

Immune-related toxicities can affect several organs. In the following, the epidemiology, diagnosis, and management of immune-related adverse event are reviewed by organ system.

## SKIN TOXICITIES

Skin toxicity is the most common immune-related adverse event observed with ICI. Forty percent of patients treated with ipilimumab experience cutaneous adverse effects. These toxicities are dose dependent with dermatologic toxicity occurring more frequently at the higher dose of 10 mg/kg compared with the lower dose of 3 mg/kg.[18] Cutaneous adverse events usually occur within 3 to 6 weeks after starting ipilimumab, but can arise at any time during the course of treatment or after treatment cessation.[19] The most common dermatologic toxicity is a morbilliform rash, which typically spares the head, palms, and soles.[19] Pruritus without a rash can also occur. Other less common side effects include lichenoid eruptions, prurigo nodularis, pyoderma gangrenosum, sweet syndrome, bullous dermatoses, and cutaneous sarcoidosis.[19]

Cutaneous adverse events are similar with PD-1 and PD-L1 inhibitors but typically arise later in the course of treatment compared with CTLA-4 inhibitors, ranging from 2 to 10 months.[19] A systematic review showed the incidence of pruritus ranged from 2.3% to 31.7% with nivolumab and 10% to 25.8% with pembrolizumab.[20] The rash from PD-1 and PD-L1 inhibitors is typically maculopapular, similar to that seen with CTLA-4 inhibition. Histologic examination of skin biopsies typically reveals a dermal hypersensitivity reaction with perivascular lymphocytic infiltrates and eosinophils.[18]

Management of mild, inflammatory rashes that do not affect quality of life involves topical corticosteroids with continuation of treatment. For grade 2 rashes, which affect quality of life, a treatment hold should be considered and oral corticosteroids can be used. Rashes are defined as grade 3 if they fail to respond to treatment. Treatment for grade 3 involves higher-dose corticosteroids. Grade 4 disease is defined as severe rashes that are intolerable and not improved with prior interventions. Treatment of grade 4 rashes includes inpatient admission with intravenous (IV) corticosteroids.[21]

Vitiligo, which is characterized by depigmented macules and patches, can occur with the use of ICIs to treat melanoma. In clinical trials of PD-1 and PD-L1 inhibitors in the treatment of melanoma, the incidence of vitiligo was 7.5% with nivolumab and 8.3% with pembrolizumab.[20] Vitiligo typically occurs several months after the initiation of treatment, which is later than other cutaneous side effects often observed.[21] It typically persists after discontinuation or completion of treatment and can become coalescent over time.[12] In a retrospective study of melanoma patients receiving nivolumab, vitiligo was observed in 9.6% of patients with metastatic disease and 24.2% of patients with resected disease. Development of vitiligo in patients with resected and metastatic melanoma is associated with a statistically significant improvement in overall survival (hazard ratio [HR], 0.22; 95% confidence interval [CI] 0.025–0.806; $P = .028$).[12] A meta-analysis of vitiligo in melanoma patients receiving various types of immunotherapy, including ICIs, vaccines, adoptive transfer, and immune stimulation, revealed a 4-fold improvement in overall survival (HR, 0.25; 95% CI, 0.10–0.61; $P<.003$) compared with patients who did not develop vitiligo.[14]

## GASTROINTESTINAL TOXICITIES

Gastrointestinal toxicities are the second most common immune-related adverse event after dermatologic side effects. Patients can develop inflammation of any part of the gastrointestinal tract, with involvement of the colon (colitis) being the most common.

### Colitis

Diarrhea is a frequent side effect of ICIs and has been reported in up to 44% of patients after treatment with the combination of CTLA-4 and PD-1 inhibition, 35% after CTLA-4 inhibition alone, and 20% after PD-1 inhibition alone.[22] Timely diagnosis of colitis in a patient who develops diarrhea after ICI is critical, but can be challenging. Typically, there are signs of colitis on computed tomographic (CT) scan, or endoscopy shows characteristic inflammation with evidence of colitis on pathology.[23] In one study of ICI-induced diarrhea/colitis, 50% of patients had concurrent abdominal pain and 30% had hematochezia.[22] Although colitis is often mild, it can be severe and lead to intestinal perforation or death.[24] The incidence of colitis and timing of onset vary based on the type of ICI used. Colitis occurs more often with the use of ipilimumab and most frequently with the combination of ipilimumab/nivolumab treatment. In a recent meta-analysis of more than 8000 patients on prospective clinical trials of ICIs, the incidence of all-grade colitis was 13.6% with combination ipilimumab/nivolumab, 9.1% with ipilimumab, 1.4% with nivolumab, and 1.0% with atezolizumab.[25] Diarrhea develops at a median of 30 days with the use of combination ipilimumab/nivolumab therapy or ipilimumab alone and can manifest later with the use of PD-1 antibodies up to a median of 84 days after the initiation of treatment.[22] The incidence of grade 3 to 4 gastrointestinal side effects is dose related and reported to be 0%, 3%, and 15% in patients receiving 0.3, 3, and 10 mg/kg of ipilimumab, respectively.[24]

Endoscopic evaluation of patients with colitis often shows erythema, edema, loss of vascular patterns, erosions, or ulceration similar to that seen in inflammatory bowel disease.[26] The inflammation is usually continuous, but can be patchy.[24,26] Disease can occur in any part of the gastrointestinal tract, including the esophagus, stomach, small bowel, and colon.[26] If endoscopy shows ulceration, pancolitis, or a higher Mayo endoscopic score, which is used to monitor disease activity in ulcerative colitis, there is an increased risk of steroid-refractory colitis, which then requires second-line immunosuppressive treatments, such as infliximab.[22,24] For evaluation, a rectosigmoidoscopy is usually sufficient because disease most often affects the descending colon. However, if the left side does not show severe disease, a full colonoscopy is recommended because the ascending colon can be affected.

Biopsy often shows acute colitis, which is characterized by focal active colitis with patchy crypt abscess formation or diffuse mucosal inflammation[26] (**Fig. 1**). In one study of ipilimumab-induced colitis, biopsies showed infiltration of neutrophils in 46%, lymphocytes in 15%, and mixed neutrophil and lymphocyte in 38%. Granulomas are rarely seen.[26,27]

Although colonoscopy with biopsy is the gold standard for diagnosing colitis, CT scan has been shown to be a fast, noninvasive, diagnostic tool (**Fig. 2**). In a retrospective study of patients who developed diarrhea while receiving ipilimumab, CT scan had a positive predictive value of 96% when compared with biopsy-proven disease.[28] This study suggests that CT scan can be used to make a diagnosis of colitis but cannot rule out disease, and further workup should be obtained in the case of a negative CT scan.

In cases of suspected colitis, infection and hyperthyroidism should be ruled out and treatment should be initiated promptly. Grade 1 colitis, defined as an increase of fewer than 4 stools per day, can be monitored closely with continuation of treatment. For grade 2 through 4 disease, treatment should be held, corticosteroids initiated, and endoscopy pursued. If symptoms continue despite corticosteroids or symptoms improve and then recur, IV corticosteroids and infliximab therapy should be considered.[21]

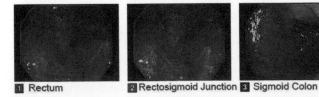 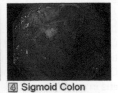

1 Rectum    2 Rectosigmoid Junction  3 Sigmoid Colon    4 Sigmoid Colon

**Fig. 1.** Colonoscopy findings in a patient with colitis demonstrating erythema and erosions.

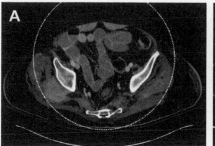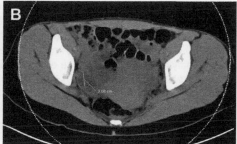

**Fig. 2.** (*A, B*) CT imaging from 2 patients with colitis demonstrating fluid-filled loops and stranding adjacent to bowel.

There have been efforts at trying to prevent colitis. Budesonide, which is a nonabsorbed oral steroid, has been evaluated in a prophylactic manner. A randomized, double-blind, placebo-controlled trial of prophylactic budesonide in melanoma patients receiving ipilimumab did not show any benefit to prophylaxis because there were similar rates of diarrhea and colitis in both arms.[29]

### Hepatitis

Hepatic toxicity manifests as hepatitis with hepatocellular injury and elevation in serum aspartate aminotransferase (AST), alanine aminotransferase (ALT), and (sometimes) bilirubin.[24] Hepatitis is often asymptomatic; however, patients can develop nausea, vomiting, or abdominal pain.[30] Hepatic toxicity can occur at any time but most commonly develops about 6 to 14 weeks after initiation of treatment.

Blood tests for autoimmune liver disease are usually negative.[24] The most common finding on liver biopsy is panlobular hepatitis followed by acinar zone 3 hepatitis.[30] An inflammatory infiltrate of lymphocytes and histiocytes in a mainly sinusoidal distribution is seen. Lymphocytic infiltrates are mainly composed of CD8[+] T cells with some CD4[+] T cells and scattered CD20[+] B cells.[30]

Hepatitis usually resolves with the use of corticosteroids alone, but occasionally requires additional immunosuppressive therapy.[24] Grade 1 disease with mild increase in serum aminotransferases and bilirubin can be monitored closely without intervention. For grade 2 disease, defined by an increase in AST or ALT 3 to 5 times the upper limit of normal (ULN) and/or an increase in total bilirubin of 1.5 to 3 times the ULN, treatment should be held and corticosteroids initiated if elevation persists. For grade 3 and 4 disease, treatment should be permanently discontinued and corticosteroids initiated promptly. If there is no improvement after 3 days of corticosteroids, use of mycophenolate mofetil or azathioprine should be considered.[21,24]

## ENDOCRINE TOXICITIES
### Thyroiditis

Alteration of thyroid function is one of the most common adverse events resulting from treatment with ICIs. Severe thyroid dysfunction is rare with a reported incidence of grade 3 hypothyroidism and hyperthyroidism of 0.2%.[31] Incidence of hypothyroidism and hyperthyroidism varies based on the type of ICI used.[31] Guidelines recommend thyroid studies (thyroid stimulating hormone [TSH] and free thyroxine [FT4]) before every treatment or at least once per month.[32] Most cases of thyroid dysfunction are diagnosed based on routine laboratory tests rather than clinical symptoms.[32] The most common clinical scenario is development of thyroiditis sometimes associated with a transient thyrotoxic phase typically followed by persistent hypothyroidism.[33]

The pathophysiology of thyroid toxicity from ICI is not completely understood. PD-L1 and PD-L2 messenger RNA is known to be expressed in normal thyroid tissue.[33] In a meta-analysis of 38 prospective clinical trials of ICIs, the overall incidence of hypothyroidism was 3.8% with CTLA-4 inhibition, 7.0% with PD-1 inhibition, 3.9% with PD-L1 inhibition, and 13.2% with combination CTLA-4 and PD-1 inhibition.[31] Patients who received treatment with PD-1 or combination therapy were more likely to experience hypothyroidism than with ipilimumab alone (odds ratio [OR] 1.89; 95% CI, 1.17–3.05; adjusted $P = .03$).

Management of hypothyroidism involves thyroid hormone supplementation. For grade 1 disease with a TSH less than 10 and no symptoms, patients can continue to be monitored closely without thyroid hormone supplementation. For any symptoms of hypothyroidism, a TSH persistently greater than 10 and a low T4, thyroid hormone supplementation should be started and treatment can be held until symptoms resolve or continued if symptoms are mild. For severe cases with symptoms of myxedema, patients should be admitted for IV therapy and close monitoring.[21]

The incidence of hyperthyroidism is lower than that of hypothyroidism. A meta-analysis reported the overall incidence of hyperthyroidism to be 1.7% with CTLA-4 inhibition, 3.2% with PD-1 inhibition, 0.6% with PD-L1 inhibition, and 8.0% with combined CTLA-4 and PD-1 inhibition. Combination therapy with CTLA-4 and PD-1 inhibitors was more likely to result in hyperthyroidism compared with treatment with ipilimumab alone (OR, 4.27; 95% CI, 2.05–8.90; $P = .001$).[31] Treatment with PD-1 inhibitors also results in a higher incidence of hyperthyroidism than PD-L1 (OR, 5.36; 95% CI, 2.04–14.08; adjusted $P = .002$). Among PD-1 inhibitors, pembrolizumab is associated with a slightly higher incidence of hyperthyroidism compared with nivolumab (3.8% [95% CI, 2.1%-6.9%] vs 2.5% [95% CI, 1.3%-4.6%], $P = .04$).[31]

For asymptomatic or mildly symptomatic hyperthyroidism, treatment can be continued with close monitoring. For grade 2 disease with moderate symptoms, treatment can be continued and patients treated supportively with beta-blockers and hydration. If hyperthyroidism persists for longer than 6 weeks, testing for Graves disease should be done with initiation of thionamide treatment if positive. For grade 3 to 4 disease, which is characterized by severe symptoms limiting daily life, treatment should be held, beta-blocker started, and corticosteroids started. The patient may also require treatment with potassium iodide or thionamide. Patients with symptoms of thyroid storm need to be hospitalized for treatment and close monitoring.[21]

### Hypophysitis

Hypophysitis consists of inflammation of the pituitary gland with alteration of hormone function. Patients who develop hypophysitis can present with headache or visual symptoms due to local effects of swelling of the pituitary gland or with nonspecific symptoms, such as fatigue, nausea, weakness, or loss of appetite from pituitary hormone dysfunction. Patients typically develop central adrenal insufficiency, and this can be accompanied by hypotension, hyponatremia, hypothyroidism, diabetes insipidus, or hypogonadism.[21] Endocrine adverse events such as hypophysitis typically occur around 9 weeks after treatment initiation but can manifest much later, over 1 year after treatment starts. Diagnostic workup should include brain MRI (**Fig. 3**) and hormonal workup, including ACTH, cortisol, TSH, FT4, T3, and others. In a meta-analysis of 6472 patients with advanced solid tumor malignancies who received ICI therapy, the incidence of any grade hypophysitis was 1.3%. Of the patients who developed hypophysitis, 89% were being treated for melanoma. Of these patients,

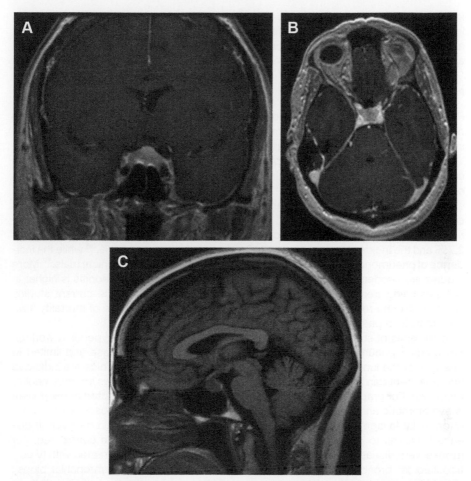

**Fig. 3.** (*A–C*) Brain imaging from a patient with hypophysitis demonstrating pituitary enlargement.

the incidence of hypophysitis was highest with combination CTLA-4 and PD-1 therapy at 6.4%, slightly lower with CTLA-4 treatment alone at 3.2%, and lowest with PD-1 inhibitors at 0.4% and PD-L1 inhibitors at less than 0.1%.[31]

Evaluation of the cause of hypophysitis has demonstrated CTLA-4 expression on a subset of adenohypophyseal endocrine cells. CTLA-4 expression occurs at different levels in different individuals and is thought to be responsible for the hypophysitis observed with ipilimumab.[34] Patients who develop hypophysitis typically require life-long corticosteroid replacement. High doses of steroids during the development of hypophysitis have not been demonstrated to rescue endocrine function.

Patients need corticosteroid replacement as well as thyroid and hormonal replacement if indicated based on testing. Corticosteroids should always be given for several days before thyroid replacement to avoid adrenal crisis.[21]

### Rare Endocrine Adverse Events

ICIs can rarely cause other endocrine toxicities, such as primary adrenal insufficiency and autoimmune diabetes mellitus. In a meta-analysis of 62 studies, primary adrenal insufficiency was seen in 0.7% of patients and insulin-dependent diabetes developed in 0.2%.[31] Primary adrenal insufficiency warrants corticosteroid replacement therapy and may require fludrocortisone for mineralocorticoid replacement. Development of autoimmune diabetes should be treated with insulin as type 1 diabetes.[21]

## PULMONARY TOXICITIES

Pneumonitis can occur with ICI, and its presentation can vary in severity; rarely, it can be a life-threatening adverse event. Time to onset of pneumonitis typically occurs several weeks after initiating treatment.[35]

Patients with pneumonitis can present with new respiratory symptoms, such as cough, dyspnea, or hypoxia. Imaging often shows bilateral, peripheral ground glass or consolidative opacities[35] (**Fig. 4**).

Pneumonitis is much more common in patients treated with PD-1 inhibitors compared with a CTLA-4 inhibitor. In a retrospective review of more than 4000 patients treated with a PD-1 inhibitor, the incidence of any grade pneumonitis was 2.7% and the incidence of severe grade 3 or higher disease was 0.8%,[36] while the incidence of pneumonitis after CTLA-4 inhibition was less than 1% in clinical trials.[17] More studies are needed to determine whether the rate of severe pneumonitis is higher in patients being treated for a diagnosis of lung cancer because the current studies show conflicting results.[35,36] There does appear to be a higher rate of mortality from pneumonitis in patients with lung cancer.[35]

In all cases of suspected pneumonitis, treatment should be held pending workup. For grade 1 pneumonitis, which is defined as asymptomatic disease and limited to one lobe of the lung or less than 25% of lung parenchyma, no steroids are indicated and treatment can be resumed if repeat testing in 3 to 4 weeks shows improvement or resolution. For grade 2 disease, in which 25% to 50% of lung is affected or the patient is symptomatic and limited in some activities of daily living, bronchoscopy with bronchoalveolar lavage (BAL) should be done and corticosteroids should be given. If disease improves to grade 1 or resolves, restarting treatment can be considered. For more severe disease classified as grade 3 or 4, patients should be treated with IV corticosteroids; bronchoscopy with BAL should be performed; transbronchial biopsy should be considered, and treatment should be permanently discontinued. If there

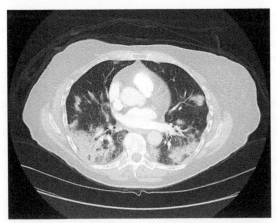

**Fig. 4.** Pulmonary imaging from a patient with pneumonitis demonstrating bilateral diffuse opacities.

is no clinical improvement after 48 hours, additional immunosuppressive therapy, such as infliximab, mycophenolate mofetil, IV immunoglobulin, or cyclophosphamide, should be considered.[21]

## NEUROLOGIC TOXICITIES

Neurologic immune-related adverse events are uncommon but potentially serious. The most common neurologic side effects are mild, including headache or peripheral sensory neuropathy. Toxicities can vary depending on the immunotherapy agent used. In an analysis of 1500 patients with melanoma treated with ipilimumab, neurologic adverse events were seen in 0.1% of patients.[37] Treatment with ipilimumab has been rarely associated with peripheral neuropathy, Guillain-Barre syndrome, myasthenia gravis, aseptic meningitis, and chronic inflammatory demyelinating polyneuropathy.[37] Neurologic toxicity is less common with PD-1 inhibitors. Adverse events reported include peripheral neuropathy, Guillain-Barre syndrome, and myasthenia gravis. Treatment with nivolumab has also been associated with dizziness, nerve paresis, demyelination, and autoimmune neuropathy, whereas treatment with pembrolizumab has been associated with partial seizures. Immune-mediated encephalitis has also been reported and can be fatal.[37]

A review of serious neurologic immune-related adverse events in more than 3700 melanoma patients receiving nivolumab or combination of ipilimumab and nivolumab on a clinical trial from 2008 to 2016 was conducted. Serious events were defined as those considered medically significant, life threatening, requiring hospitalization, or resulting in disability or death. Of patients, 0.93% were reported to have developed a serious neurologic toxicity potentially related to their immunotherapy treatment. The most common neurologic adverse events were neuropathy (63%), encephalitis (17%), aseptic meningitis (14%), neuromuscular disorders (9%), and nonspecific events (20%) with some patients experiencing more than one event. Nonspecific events included headache, seizure, confusion, and syncope. Out of a total of 43 events, there was 1 case of fatal encephalitis. The time to onset of neurologic adverse events was a median of 45 days with a range of 1 to 170 days.[37]

### Encephalitis

Patients with immune-related encephalitis can present with altered mental status characterized by confusion, aphasia, or agitation; ataxia; seizure; or fatigue. Treatment includes antiviral therapy and antibiotics to cover viral and bacterial encephalitis until an infectious cause is excluded. Management of immune-mediated encephalitis should include IV corticosteroids and treatment should be discontinued. Immunoglobulins or other immunosuppressive medications should be considered.

## CARDIOVASCULAR TOXICITIES

Immune-related adverse events include cardiac toxicity in the form of myocarditis, pericarditis, or cardiomyopathy. Although cardiomyopathy is a rare side effect seen in less than 1% of patients, it can be serious or even fatal. Symptoms of cardiomyopathy are nonspecific and can include chest pain, shortness of breath, and fatigue. The pathophysiology is not clearly known. Studies have shown that human and murine hearts express PD-L1.[38] It has been demonstrated that mice lacking PD-1 develop dilated cardiomyopathy and congestive heart failure.[39] Affected mice have a high titer of circulating immunoglobulin G (IgG) autoantibodies against a protein on cardiomyocyte surface, and autopsies showed linear deposition of IgG on cardiomyocytes in PD-1–deficient mice but not in normal mice.[39]

Myocarditis is a rare but serious immune-related adverse event. In a review of more than 20,000 patients who were treated with ipilimumab, nivolumab, or the combination of both, 0.09% of patients experienced myocarditis. The average time to onset of myocarditis was 17 days, ranging from 13 to 64 days. Myocarditis was rare with any of the treatments; it occurred more frequently with the combination of ipilimumab and nivolumab compared with nivolumab alone, 0.27% versus 0.06%, respectively.[40] In 2 case reports of fatal myocarditis in clinical trials, the patients developed complete heart block and cardiac arrest. Autopsies of these patients showed immune cell infiltration of cardiac skeletal muscle, cardiac sinus, and the atrioventricular node.[40]

Management of myocarditis, pericarditis, or cardiomyopathy includes consideration of permanent treatment discontinuation at all grades. Patients should be treated promptly with high-dose glucocorticoids with further interventions guided by cardiology consultation.[21,40] If patients do not respond quickly to high-dose corticosteroids, pulse dose methylprednisolone at 1000 mg daily per cardiac transplant rejection treatment and consideration of mycophenolate mofetil, infliximab, or antithymocyte globulin should be considered. Infliximab should not be used at high doses in patients with moderate to severe heart failure given the drug's association with heart failure itself.[21]

## RENAL TOXICITIES

ICIs can rarely cause renal toxicity. In a review of more than 3600 patients enrolled in phase 2 and 3 clinical trials of ICI, the incidence of acute kidney injury (AKI) was 2.2% overall with an incidence of grade III or IV renal disease of 0.6%.[41] The incidence of AKI varied between treatment regimens and was reported at 4.9% with combination ipilimumab-nivolumab, 2.0% with ipilimumab, 1.9% with nivolumab, and 1.4% with pembrolizumab.[41] Development of AKI ranged in onset from 21 to 245 days with a median of 91 days after the start of immunotherapy treatment.[41]

In a case series of 13 patients who developed renal toxicity after receiving an ICI and underwent a renal biopsy, the most common pathologic condition seen was acute tubulointerstitial nephritis (AIN). In the case of AIN, biopsies showed a lymphocytic infiltrate with a predominance of CD3$^+$ T lymphocytes. Granulomas were seen in 3 cases.[41]

The mechanism of AKI development after ICIs is not known, but it is thought to be separate from a typical drug-induced AIN. The delayed onset after drug initiation supports an immune-related cause. It is hypothesized that CTLA-4 and PD-1 inhibitors cause a loss of tolerance to endogenous antigens present in the kidney leading to an immune infiltrate and development of AIN.[41]

Patients who develop renal toxicity are commonly asymptomatic and present with an elevated creatinine detected on routine laboratory tests. In the above described case series of 13 patients who developed AKI after receiving an ICI, peak creatinine ranged from 2.5 to 13.3 with a median of 4.5.[41] Two patients presented with new onset hypertension; 2 patients developed oliguria, and pyuria was seen in 8 cases and hematuria in 3 cases. Mild proteinuria was seen with a urine protein:creatinine ratio ranging from 0.12 to 0.98 g/g. Seven of the 13 patients had a preceding diagnosis of an immune-related adverse event in another organ system.[41] Of 10 patients with biopsy-proven AIN who received corticosteroids for treatment, 2 patients recovered renal function to baseline and 7 patients partially recovered renal function. Two patients with biopsy-proven AIN were not treated with corticosteroids and did not recover renal function. Treatment was initially discontinued in all cases. However, treatment was resumed in 2 cases after improvement in renal function, and these patients did not develop recurrent renal injury. Two of the 13 patients required temporary dialysis and another 2 patients required long-term dialysis.[41]

If nephritis is suspected, treatment should be held pending further evaluation. For a creatinine 2 to 3 times above baseline, corticosteroids should be initiated and high-dose corticosteroids used if there is no improvement. For a creatinine greater than 3 times baseline or requiring dialysis, treatment should be permanently discontinued.[21]

## RHEUMATOLOGIC/MUSCULOSKELETAL TOXICITIES

Arthralgias and myalgias are relatively common musculoskeletal adverse events seen with ICIs.

### *Arthralgia/Arthritis*

Arthralgias and arthritis are thought to be underestimated adverse events associated with ICIs. The incidence of arthralgias is reported to range from 5% to 16% in phase 3 trials of the PD-1 antibody, nivolumab.[42] A systematic review of 52 articles including musculoskeletal and rheumatic adverse events found that the prevalence of arthralgias in clinical trials ranged from 1% to 43%.[43] The incidence of inflammatory arthritis is not well known because it is often reported under arthralgia. In a meta-analysis of 5 clinical trials that reported on arthritis, the incidence ranged from 1% to 7%.[43] Arthritis is characterized by joint pain with associated swelling, stiffness after activity, or improvement in symptoms with nonsteroidal anti-inflammatory drugs (NSAIDs) or corticosteroids.[21] Patients typically experience bilateral pain of the large joints alone, such as shoulders and knees. Less frequently, symptoms also involve joints of the feet and wrists, whereas finger joints, spine, elbows, and hips are affected rarely. Patients do not typically have symptoms in small joints alone without involvement of large joints.[44] Most patients with arthritis test negative for rheumatoid factor and anticyclic citrullinated peptide.[42,44]

In a retrospective study of 195 patients receiving anti-PD-1 therapy, the incidence of arthralgia was 13.3% and the incidence of clinical arthritis was 0.5%. The median onset of arthralgia was 100 days (range 7–780 days) after initiating treatment. In some patients, synovitis could be seen on MRI or PET/CT, and several patients were found to have inflammation of joints with preexisting osteoarthritis.[44] Arthrocentesis done in the cases of synovitis showed inflammatory synovial fluid with 9000 to 30,000 white blood cells per milliliter with neutrophil predominance.[42] Most patients were adequately treated with NSAIDs, whereas 23% required low-dose corticosteroids and only 7.6% received additional immunosuppressive therapy.[44]

In most studies, arthritis is generally mild and grade 1 to 2. For grade 1 disease with mild symptoms, treatment can be continued and symptoms managed with NSAIDs or acetaminophen. For grade 2 disease with moderate symptoms limiting daily activities, treatment can be held and low-dose corticosteroids used if needed. For severe, grade 3 to 4 disease, corticosteroids should be used, and if unable to be tapered, then disease-modifying antirheumatic drugs should be considered.

### *Myalgia/Myositis*

Myalgias have been reported in 2% to 20% of patients on clinical trials with ICI.[43] Myositis with muscle inflammation, weakness, and elevated creatine kinase (CK) is a rare, but potentially serious immune-related adverse event. The incidence is not known, and the most information comes from case reports and case series. Myositis can be life threatening when it involves muscles of the heart or diaphragm.

In a retrospective analysis of 10 patients treated with ICIs for treatment of melanoma, lung cancer, breast cancer, or renal cell carcinoma who were diagnosed with immune related myositis, average time to onset was 25 days after initiation of therapy (range 5–87).[45] The most common symptoms were acute to subacute myalgia, limbgirdle weakness, axial weakness, and oculomotor weakness. In most patients, pain preceded the development of weakness. Limb weakness was symmetric, whereas oculomotor weakness was asymmetric in most cases. Less common symptoms included dysphonia, dyspnea, and fatigue. Symptoms are typically progressive and do not fluctuate. Almost half of the patients had preceding immune-related adverse events of other organs before the development of myositis. Myositis was grade 3 to 4 in most patients diagnosed. One patient had involvement of the diaphragm causing respiratory failure requiring intubation. Four of the patients had concurrent myocarditis, and 3 of these patients had severe, disabling myositis.[45] ICI treatment was permanently discontinued in all 10 patients. Most patients received corticosteroids, whereas one patient required methotrexate and 3 patients required IV immunoglobulin or plasma exchange. All patients experienced an improvement in their symptoms with normalization of CK levels in a median of 44 days (range 6–96).[45]

Diagnosis of myositis can be based on objective muscle weakness, elevated CK level, electrodiagnostic studies showing a myopathic process without decrementing response during repetitive nerve stimulation, or muscle biopsy showing myositis. In the case series of 10 patients with myositis, all patients had elevated CK levels with a median of 2668 U/L (range 1059–16,620 U/L) and negative anti–acetylcholine receptor antibody and negative myositis-associated antibodies.[45] Electromyography shows abnormal spontaneous movement or myopathic motor units with normal or early recruitment, characteristic of a myopathic process. This myopathic process is mainly observed in the muscles of the proximal limbs, deltoids, and trapezius. Repetitive nerve stimulation should not show a decremental response, which would be seen in neuromuscular disorders such as myasthenia gravis.[45]

Muscle biopsies done in cases of myositis show multifocal necrotic myofibers with significant infiltration of macrophages and T cells. Major histocompatibility complex-I molecules in the sarcolemma of myofibers have been identified in areas of severe necrosis indicating an inflammatory myopathy. Focal inflammatory infiltrates in the endomysium consist of CD68$^+$ cells, CD8$^+$ cells, CD4$^+$ cells, and rare CD20$^+$ cells. PD-1 expression has been identified on T cells seen diffusely as well as surrounding myofiber necrosis but not invading the myofibers. PD-L1 has been observed on macrophages. Because of the focal nature of the infiltrates, site of muscle biopsy should be chosen based on location of clinical, electrophysiologic, or radiographic abnormalities.[45]

Guidelines for treatment of myositis classify mild muscle weakness with or without pain and no CK elevation as grade 1. Treatment can be continued and symptoms managed with NSAIDs or acetaminophen. For grade 2 disease with moderate symptoms limiting daily activity, treatment should be held and corticosteroids initiated for CK elevation. Permanent treatment discontinuation should be considered for patients with grade 2 disease, CK elevation, and testing consistent with myositis. For severe, grade 3 to 4 disease, high-dose corticosteroids should be used, and additional treatment such as plasmapheresis, IV immunoglobulin, methotrexate, azathioprine, mycophenolate mofetil, or rituximab should be considered.[21]

## PREEXISTENT AUTOIMMUNE DISEASES

One of the concerns with immune-associated toxicity is that patients with baseline autoimmune disease may experience worse toxicity. Clinical trials previously excluded these patients from enrollment. However, series of patients treated with immunotherapy have demonstrated that these agents can be administered relatively safely to most patients with preexistent autoimmune diseases, but patients need to be watched closely for toxicity.[46,47]

## FUTURE DIRECTIONS

Work to better understand and limit the incidence of immune-related toxicities is ongoing. One study evaluating the efficacy of adding granulocyte-macrophage colony-stimulating factor (GM-CSF) to ipilimumab versus ipilimumab alone for treatment of melanoma showed an improvement in overall survival (17.5 vs 12.7 months, $P = .01$) as well as a lower occurrence of grade 3 to 5 serious adverse events (44.9% vs 58.3%, $P = .04$).[48] This study showed lower rates of serious gastrointestinal toxicity with GM-CSF (16.1% vs 26.7%), including fewer colonic perforations as well as less pulmonary toxicity (0% vs 7.5%).[48] Studies such as these may provide insight into agents that can be safely given to limit toxicity without affecting the anticancer immune effect.

As immunotherapy becomes more widely used, structured management approaches and national guidelines are being put in place to formally guide toxicity management. The American Society of Clinical Oncology, National Comprehensive Cancer Network, Society of Immunotherapy of Cancer, and European Society for Medical Oncology have published management guidelines.[21,32,49,50] In addition, close collaborations are being established between oncology providers and physicians with organ system expertise to establish management plans appropriate for the site of toxicity. Many centers have established institutional guidelines, toxicity algorithms, and multidisciplinary teams to assist with immunotoxicity management.

Further studies are ongoing to better understand immune-related adverse events with goals of reducing the incidence and improving the treatment of these side effects. This work will also contribute to a better understanding of autoimmune diseases and the immune system as a whole.

## REFERENCES

1. Hodi FS, O'Day SJ, McDermott DF, et al. Improved survival with ipilimumab in patients with metastatic melanoma. N Engl J Med 2010;363(8):711–23.
2. Topalian SL, Hodi FS, Brahmer JR, et al. Safety, activity, and immune correlates of anti-PD-1 antibody in cancer. N Engl J Med 2012;366(26):2443–54.
3. Topalian SL, Sznol M, McDermott DF, et al. Survival, durable tumor remission, and long-term safety in patients with advanced melanoma receiving nivolumab. J Clin Oncol 2014;32(10):1020–30.
4. Robert C, Schachter J, Long GV, et al. Pembrolizumab versus ipilimumab in advanced melanoma. N Engl J Med 2015;372(26):2521–32.
5. Motzer RJ, Escudier B, McDermott DF, et al. Nivolumab versus Everolimus in advanced renal-cell carcinoma. N Engl J Med 2015;373(19):1803–13.
6. Herbst RS, Soria JC, Kowanetz M, et al. Predictive correlates of response to the anti-PD-L1 antibody MPDL3280A in cancer patients. Nature 2014;515(7528): 563–7.
7. Larkin J, Chiarion-Sileni V, Gonzalez R, et al. Combined nivolumab and ipilimumab or monotherapy in untreated melanoma. N Engl J Med 2015;373(1):23–34.
8. Goldrath AW, Bevan MJ. Selecting and maintaining a diverse T-cell repertoire. Nature 1999;402(6759):255–62.
9. Fife BT, Bluestone JA. Control of peripheral T-cell tolerance and autoimmunity via the CTLA-4 and PD-1 pathways. Immunol Rev 2008;224:166–82.

10. Amos SM, Duong CP, Westwood JA, et al. Autoimmunity associated with immunotherapy of cancer. Blood 2011;118(3):499–509.
11. Bertrand A, Kostine M, Barnetche T, et al. Immune related adverse events associated with anti-CTLA-4 antibodies: systematic review and meta-analysis. BMC Med 2015;13:211.
12. Freeman-Keller M, Kim Y, Cronin H, et al. Nivolumab in resected and unresectable metastatic melanoma: characteristics of immune-related adverse events and association with outcomes. Clin Cancer Res 2016;22(4):886–94.
13. Nakamura Y, Tanaka R, Asami Y, et al. Correlation between vitiligo occurrence and clinical benefit in advanced melanoma patients treated with nivolumab: a multi-institutional retrospective study. J Dermatol 2017;44(2):117–22.
14. Teulings HE, Limpens J, Jansen SN, et al. Vitiligo-like depigmentation in patients with stage III-IV melanoma receiving immunotherapy and its association with survival: a systematic review and meta-analysis. J Clin Oncol 2015;33(7):773–81.
15. Weber JS, Kahler KC, Hauschild A. Management of immune-related adverse events and kinetics of response with ipilimumab. J Clin Oncol 2012;30(21):2691–7.
16. D'Angelo SP, Larkin J, Sosman JA, et al. Efficacy and safety of Nivolumab alone or in combination with ipilimumab in patients with mucosal melanoma: a pooled analysis. J Clin Oncol 2017;35(2):226–35.
17. Wolchok JD, Neyns B, Linette G, et al. Ipilimumab monotherapy in patients with pretreated advanced melanoma: a randomised, double-blind, multicentre, phase 2, dose-ranging study. Lancet Oncol 2010;11(2):155–64.
18. Curry JL, Tetzlaff MT, Nagarajan P, et al. Diverse types of dermatologic toxicities from immune checkpoint blockade therapy. J Cutan Pathol 2017;44(2):158–76.
19. Collins LK, Chapman MS, Carter JB, et al. Cutaneous adverse effects of the immune checkpoint inhibitors. Curr Probl Cancer 2017;41(2):125–8.
20. Belum VR, Benhuri B, Postow MA, et al. Characterisation and management of dermatologic adverse events to agents targeting the PD-1 receptor. Eur J Cancer 2016;60:12–25.
21. Brahmer JR, Lacchetti C, Schneider BJ, et al. Management of immune-related adverse events in patients treated with immune checkpoint inhibitor therapy: American Society of Clinical oncology clinical practice guideline. J Clin Oncol 2018;36(17):1714–68.
22. Geukes Foppen MH, Rozeman EA, van Wilpe S, et al. Immune checkpoint inhibition-related colitis: symptoms, endoscopic features, histology and response to management. ESMO Open 2018;3(1):e000278.
23. Prieux-Klotz C, Dior M, Damotte D, et al. Immune checkpoint inhibitor-induced colitis: diagnosis and management. Target Oncol 2017;12(3):301–8.
24. Reddy HG, Schneider BJ, Tai AW. Immune checkpoint inhibitor-associated colits and hepatitis. Clin Transl Gastroenterol 2018;9(9):180.
25. Wang DY, Ye F, Zhao S, et al. Incidence of immune checkpoint inhibitor-related colitis in solid tumor patients: a systematic review and meta-analysis. Oncoimmunology 2017;6(10):e1344805.
26. Samaan MA, Pavlidis P, Papa S, et al. Gastrointestinal toxicity of immune checkpoint inhibitors: from mechanisms to management. Nat Rev Gastroenterol Hepatol 2018;15(4):222–34.
27. Beck KE, Blansfield JA, Tran KQ, et al. Enterocolitis in patients with cancer after antibody blockade of cytotoxic T-lymphocyte-associated antigen 4. J Clin Oncol 2006;24(15):2283–9.

28. Garcia-Neuer M, Marmarelis ME, Jangi SR, et al. Diagnostic comparison of CT scans and colonoscopy for immune-related colitis in ipilimumab-treated advanced melanoma patients. Cancer Immunol Res 2017;5(4):286–91.
29. Weber J, Thompson JA, Hamid O, et al. A randomized, double-blind, placebo-controlled, phase II study comparing the tolerability and efficacy of ipilimumab administered with or without prophylactic budesonide in patients with unresectable stage III or IV melanoma. Clin Cancer Res 2009;15(17):5591–8.
30. Johncilla M, Misdraji J, Pratt DS, et al. Ipilimumab-associated hepatitis: clinico-pathologic characterization in a series of 11 cases. Am J Surg Pathol 2015; 39(8):1075–84.
31. Barroso-Sousa R, Barry WT, Garrido-Castro AC, et al. Incidence of endocrine dysfunction following the use of different immune checkpoint inhibitor regimens: a systematic review and meta-analysis. JAMA Oncol 2018;4(2):173–82.
32. Haanen JBAG, Carbonnel F, Robert C, et al, ESMO Guidelines Committee. Management of toxicities from immunotherapy: ESMO Clinical Practice Guidelines for diagnosis, treatment and follow-up. Ann Oncol 2017;28(suppl_4):iv119–42.
33. Yamauchi I, Sakane Y, Fukuda Y, et al. Clinical features of nivolumab-induced thyroiditis: a case series study. Thyroid 2017;27(7):894–901.
34. Caturegli P, Di Dalmazi G, Lombardi M, et al. Hypophysitis secondary to cytotoxic T-lymphocyte-associated protein 4 blockade: insights into pathogenesis from an autopsy series. Am J Pathol 2016;186(12):3225–35.
35. Friedman CF, Proverbs-Singh TA, Postow MA. Treatment of the immune-related adverse effects of immune checkpoint inhibitors: a review. JAMA Oncol 2016; 2(10):1346–53.
36. Nishino M, Hatabu H. Programmed death-1/programmed death ligand-1 inhibitor-related pneumonitis and radiographic patterns. J Clin Oncol 2017;35(14): 1628–9.
37. Larkin J, Chmielowski B, Lao CD, et al. Neurologic serious adverse events associated with nivolumab plus ipilimumab or nivolumab alone in advanced melanoma, including a case series of encephalitis. Oncologist 2017;22(6):709–18.
38. Koga N, Suzuki J, Kosuge H, et al. Blockade of the interaction between PD-1 and PD-L1 accelerates graft arterial disease in cardiac allografts. Arterioscler Thromb Vasc Biol 2004;24(11):2057–62.
39. Nishimura H, Okazaki T, Tanaka Y, et al. Autoimmune dilated cardiomyopathy in PD-1 receptor-deficient mice. Science 2001;291(5502):319–22.
40. Johnson DB, Balko JM, Compton ML, et al. Fulminant myocarditis with combination immune checkpoint blockade. N Engl J Med 2016;375(18):1749–55.
41. Cortazar FB, Marrone KA, Troxell ML, et al. Clinicopathological features of acute kidney injury associated with immune checkpoint inhibitors. Kidney Int 2016; 90(3):638–47.
42. Cappelli LC, Shah AA, Bingham CO 3rd. Immune-related adverse effects of cancer immunotherapy- implications for rheumatology. Rheum Dis Clin North Am 2017;43(1):65–78.
43. Cappelli LC, Gutierrez AK, Bingham CO 3rd, et al. Rheumatic and musculoskeletal immune-related adverse events due to immune checkpoint inhibitors: a systematic review of the literature. Arthritis Care Res (Hoboken) 2017;69(11): 1751–63.
44. Buder-Bakhaya K, Benesova K, Schulz C, et al. Characterization of arthralgia induced by PD-1 antibody treatment in patients with metastasized cutaneous malignancies. Cancer Immunol Immunother 2018;67(2):175–82.

45. Touat M, Maisonobe T, Knauss S, et al. Immune checkpoint inhibitor-related myositis and myocarditis in patients with cancer. Neurology 2018;91(10): e985-94.
46. Menzies AM, Johnson DB, Ramanujam S, et al. Anti-PD-1 therapy in patients with advanced melanoma and preexisting autoimmune disorders or major toxicity with ipilimumab. Ann Oncol 2017;28(2):368-76.
47. Johnson DB, Sullivan RJ, Ott PA, et al. Ipilimumab therapy in patients with advanced melanoma and preexisting autoimmune disorders. JAMA Oncol 2016;2(2):234-40.
48. Hodi FS, Lee S, McDermott DF, et al. Ipilimumab plus sargramostim vs ipilimumab alone for treatment of metastatic melanoma: a randomized clinical trial. JAMA 2014;312(17):1744-53.
49. Thompson JA. New NCCN guidelines: recognition and management of immunotherapy-related toxicity. J Natl Compr Canc Netw 2018;16(5S):594-6.
50. Puzanov I, Diab A, Abdallah K, et al. Managing toxicities associated with immune checkpoint inhibitors: consensus recommendations from the Society for Immunotherapy of Cancer (SITC) Toxicity Management Working Group. J Immunother Cancer 2017;5(1):95.

# Prognostic and Predictive Immunohistochemistry-Based Biomarkers in Cancer and Immunotherapy

Emanuelle M. Rizk, BA[a], Robyn D. Gartrell, MD[a],
Luke W. Barker, BS[b], Camden L. Esancy, MS[a],
Grace G. Finkel, BA[b], Darius D. Bordbar, BS[b],
Yvonne M. Saenger, MD[a],*

## KEYWORDS

- Immunotherapy • Predictive and prognostic biomarkers • Checkpoint inhibition
- Immunohistochemistry

## KEY POINTS

- Immunotherapy has successfully improved the prognosis of patients with cancer, but its use must be closely monitored for severe immune-related adverse events.
- Predictive and prognostic biomarkers allow clinicians to weigh the potential benefits of immunotherapy against its potential toxicities by stratifying patients into risk groups.
- Immunohistochemistry (IHC) is a powerful tool for the discovery and use of biomarkers, but current techniques are limited due to lack of reproducibility.
- The combination of IHC with genomic and transcriptomic analyses and the use of multiplexed and automated IHC both may help accelerate the discovery and validation of biomarkers.

## INTRODUCTION

Over the past decade, immunotherapy has revolutionized the treatment of cancer. Immunotherapies targeted to immune checkpoint molecules, such as programmed cell death protein 1 (PD-1) and cytotoxic T-lymphocyte–associated protein 4 (CTLA-4), have significantly improved the prognosis of patients with a variety of cancers.[1] The

Disclosure Statement: The authors disclose no potential conflicts of interest.
[a] Department of Medicine, Columbia University Irving Medical Center, 650 West 168th Street, Black Building 8-816, New York, NY 10032, USA; [b] College of Physicians and Surgeons, Columbia University Irving Medical Center, 650 West 168th Street, Black Building 8-816, New York, NY 10032, USA
* Corresponding author.
E-mail address: yms4@cumc.columbia.edu

discovery of CTLA-4's function as an inhibitory molecule expressed on T cells in 1994[2,3] and the subsequent success of CTLA-4 checkpoint inhibition in clinical trials[4–8] led to the Food and Drug Administration's (FDA) approval of ipilimumab for the treatment of melanoma in 2011. More recently, inhibition of PD-1 and programmed death-ligand 1 (PD-L1) has been found to lead to durable tumor regression and prolonged disease stabilization in many types of solid tumors, including melanoma, non–small cell lung cancer (NSCLC), and renal-cell cancer.[9–11] Two PD-1 inhibitors (nivolumab and pembrolizumab) and 3 PD-L1 inhibitors (atezolizumab, durvalumab, and avelumab) have been approved by the FDA for the treatment of various cancers.[12] Finally, combined immune checkpoint blockade using nivolumab and ipilimumab has shown clinical efficacy in multiple cancer types.[13,14]

The use of immune checkpoint inhibitors must be closely monitored for severe immune-related adverse events,[15] because treatment with immune checkpoint blockade is associated with 10% to 20% grade 3 or 4 toxicities.[16] From a clinical perspective, then, the development of biomarkers to predict clinical response is critical to helping clinicians weigh the potential benefits of immunotherapy against its potential toxicities. Biomarkers may also accelerate the development of other immunotherapeutic therapies by identifying subpopulations in which these drugs would be most effective, thus allowing for clinical trial enrichment strategies.[17]

Biomarkers are biological indicators that can be subdivided into 2 categories: prognostic and predictive.[18] Although a prognostic biomarker indicates a patient's disease outcome without treatment, a predictive biomarker indicates how a patient will respond to a given therapy and may itself be a target for therapy.[19] Thus, a prognostic biomarker may help identify patients whose disease is high risk and who would benefit from aggressive therapy; a predictive biomarker may help identify patients who will benefit from a specific therapy.

In order to be effective and practical in the clinic setting, a biomarker must be both specific and sensitive, but must also be easy to use and cost-effective.[20] Because it allows for assessment of the tumor immune microenvironment and is readily applied in the clinic, immunohistochemistry (IHC) has proven to be a powerful tool for the discovery and use of biomarkers.[21–23] However, many IHC-based biomarkers have struggled to reach the clinic for a variety of reasons, in particular, due to challenges with validation or inaccuracy in predicting outcome.[24] A selection of key clinical and IHC-based biomarkers and the limitations of the use of IHC are discussed further in later discussion.

## TUMOR-INFILTRATING LYMPHOCYTES

The tumor microenvironment, composed of cell types including tumor-infiltrating lymphocytes (TILs),[25] is increasingly implicated in a bidirectional interplay with tumor cells capable of promoting or preventing tumor growth and invasion.[26] The recognition of such interactions has led to significant interest in TILs as a biomarker to both prognosticate disease outcomes and predict response to treatments such as immune checkpoint inhibitors. Early studies in primary melanoma identified the prognostic value of TILs using a classification of immune infiltrates, such as brisk, nonbrisk, or absent by conventional hematoxylin and eosin staining.[27] A higher density of TILs has been associated with favorable clinical outcomes in various cancer types, including breast cancer and melanoma.[28,29] IHC has yielded further insight into the phenotypic characterization of these immune infiltrates. As melanocytic lesions progress from benign nevi to cutaneous malignant melanomas, the absolute number of TILs increases with a relative increase in the numbers of CD3$^+$TIA-1$^+$ resting cytotoxic T lymphocytes (CTLs) as compared with CD20$^+$ B lymphocytes.[30]

In addition to its role as a prognostic biomarker, the density of TILs has also been described as a biomarker predictive of response to treatment. A 2014 study found that in HER2[+] patients with breast cancer treated with adjuvant trastuzumab, increased levels of TILs were correlated with decreased distant recurrence relative to patients receiving chemotherapy only.[31] Another study in patients with breast cancer found that density of intratumoral lymphocytes as well as protein expression of CD3, CD20, and CXCR3 is significantly associated with pathologic complete response to neoadjuvant chemotherapy.[32] Furthermore, in melanoma, CD4[+] and CD8[+] lymphocyte infiltration predicts a statistically significant favorable response to anti-PD-1 immunotherapy, underscoring the role of IHC in predicting both disease outcomes and responses to therapy.[33]

## CD8[+] TUMOR-INFILTRATING LYMPHOCYTES AND THE IMMUNOSCORE

The density of CD8[+] T cells in the tumor has been proposed as a more precise alternative to the density of TILs.[34–36] In breast cancer, the use of IHC has demonstrated that total CD8[+] lymphocytic density is an independent predictor of longer disease-specific survival, and therefore, that CD8[+] T-cell density can act as a prognostic biomarker.[35,37] In metastatic melanoma, greater numbers of CTLs with CD8 staining have been shown to correlate with longer survival,[38] a finding also demonstrated in colorectal and cervical cancer.[39,40] Furthermore, a study by Tumeh and colleagues[41] found that high density of CD8[+] TILs correlates with response to anti-PD-1 therapy in metastatic melanoma, thus suggesting that density of CD8[+] TILs may also have a role as a predictive biomarker.

As evidence increases that CD8[+] TILs confer a favorable prognosis in a variety of solid tumors, including ovarian, gallbladder, and NSCLC,[34,42,43] the Immunoscore has been proposed as a method of classifying malignant tumors by quantifying the in situ immune cell infiltrates of two lymphocyte populations.[34,42,43] In patients with colorectal cancer, the Immunoscore has been demonstrated as a biomarker with clinical utility in predicting disease recurrence following surgical resection and therefore in identifying patients likely to benefit from adjuvant therapy.[44,45] The need to reinforce the prognostic and predictive value of the Immunoscore in other solid tumors as well as to identify follow-up parameters to modify its initial prognostic value will inevitably drive further biomarker research using IHC.[46]

## PROGRAMMED CELL DEATH-1/PROGRAMMED DEATH-LIGAND 1

PD-1 and PD-L1 are immune checkpoint molecules expressed on T cells, antigen-presenting cells, and tumor cells. The presence of PD1 or PDL1 has been proposed as biomarkers predictive of response to PD-1/PD-L1 blockade. These ligands inhibit T-cell activity and are thus key to maintaining an immunosuppressed environment in the tumor. Both of these molecules are the target of several therapeutic antibodies intended to promote T-cell activity within the tumor.[47] Because most tumors do not respond to PD-1/PD-L1 inhibition, PD-1/PD-L1 expression has been investigated as a potential biomarker for response. A study in patients with NSCLC treated with pembrolizumab found that patients for whom at least 50% of tumor cells expressed PD-L1 had a response rate of 45.2%, whereas for all the patients combined the response rate was 19.4%, thus suggesting that PD-L1 expression is a predictive biomarker for response to pembrolizumab and leading to FDA approval of pembrolizumab in NSCLC in the context of tumor–PD-L1 expression as a companion biomarker.[48] Furthermore, a meta-analysis found that PD-L1 expression on tumor and tumor-infiltrating immune cells is a predictor of response across tumor types.[49] However, there remains disagreement in the field about whether PD-L1 expression alone is sufficient to accurately determine which patients will respond to checkpoint blockade. Indeed, a trial of stage III melanoma patients treated with pembrolizumab found that pembrolizumab was consistently effective both in patients with PD-L1-positive tumors and in patients with PD-L1-negative tumors, thus suggesting that PD-L1 is not a useful predictive biomarker in these patients.[50]

There are currently 4 IHC assays available to assess PD-L1 expression in patients who might be treated with anti-PD-L1 or anti-PD-1 in clinical trials. Three of these assays have shown consistency in direct comparisons, although the fourth assay indicates a lower PD-L1 expression in tumor and immune cells.[51] There are several challenges with these IHC assays, namely intratumoral heterogeneity, variable temporal expression of PD-L1, and prohibitive pricing.[52] As such, PD-L1 remains an unreliable predictive biomarker of response to PD-1/PD-L1 checkpoint inhibition.

## OTHER PREDICTIVE BIOMARKERS

Although there is no definite biomarker predicting response to CTLA-4 checkpoint inhibition, several biomarkers have been proposed for this purpose. Higher protein levels of indoleamine 2,3-dioxygenase and FoxP3 at baseline have been found to be associated with favorable clinical outcomes in patients treated with anti-CTLA-4 therapy.[53] Other studies have highlighted the importance of the ratio of effector T cells to regulatory T cells within the tumor,[54] with one study showing that the ratio of CD8+ effector T cells to FoxP3+ regulatory T cells is positively correlated with therapy-induced tumor necrosis in previously vaccinated patients with cancer treated with anti-CTLA-4.[55] Furthermore, an increase from baseline of absolute lymphocyte counts was found to positively correlate with response to anti-CTLA-4 therapy.[56] Broader changes of the immune response, such as an increase in T-cell diversity, have also been noted to follow anti-CTLA-4 immunotherapy and to be associated with a higher response rate.[57,58] Other biomarkers associated with response to anti-CTLA-4 therapy play a role only during or after treatment and, as such, cannot be used to predict response before therapy.[59]

## LIMITATIONS OF IMMUNOHISTOCHEMISTRY FOR BIOMARKER DISCOVERY AND USE

Despite IHC's ubiquitous presence in research and diagnostic procedures, it suffers from several limitations; most notably, the lack of strict guidelines for staining often results in conflicting results among different institutions using different protocols and different antibodies.[60,61] Indeed, McCabe and colleagues[60] reported that different concentrations of HER2 antibody for staining could result in opposite prognostic implications for patients with breast cancer. Beyond antibody concentration consistency, numerous other components of IHC lack quality control. For example, whether an antibody binds to its target with adequate sensitivity and specificity is not routinely tested.[62,63] The lack of staining reliability may also stem from the absence of quality control measures beyond the antibody itself. Variations in tissue fixation times, slide thickness, and antigen retrieval impact the sensitivity and specificity of the antibodies used.[64] As such, detailed and standardized protocols are necessary to allow systematic use of IHC-based biomarkers.

## FUTURE DIRECTIONS

Automated IHC platforms have the potential to improve reliability and reproducibility of IHC, which so far has limited the use of IHC-based biomarkers in the clinic. Automated

IHC platforms can be used in a clinical setting to create a "closed system" that prevents variations from being introduced.[61] Furthermore, automated image analysis platforms that decrease observer variability can more reliably quantitate biomarker positivity or negativity in patient samples.[65] However, as of yet, these platforms remain only semi-automated because they require significant input from the user to aid in the machine learning process.

Although the biomarkers described in this review have been discovered and analyzed using traditional IHC, new technologies allow for more sophisticated analyses of molecular markers. For example, technologies that allow for multiplexed immunofluorescence, such as Vectra or AQUA, allow for analysis of multiple cell phenotypes at a time.[66,67] Importantly, the multiplexing aspect of these technologies opens the possibility of evaluating the proximity between individual cells.[68] These additional dimensions of analysis may allow for further specification of a biomarker. Indeed, the authors' laboratory has recently used multiplexed immunofluorescence to find that a low CTL to macrophage ratio in the stroma is associated with lower overall survival, and that a closer distance of CTLs to HLA-DR$^-$ macrophages is associated with poor prognosis in melanoma.[66] Such biomarker discovery has been facilitated by the use of multiplexed, quantitative IHC in many other tumor types, such as breast cancer, pancreatic cancer, and squamous cell cancer.[68-70]

Finally, although biomarkers may act as independent indicators, a single biomarker is often insufficient to clearly and safely stratify patients.[71] Combining IHC with genomic and transcriptomic techniques may help in identification of more precise and predictive biomarkers, because many biomarkers have been discovered using these techniques.[72,73] For example, Hugo and colleagues[74] conducted genomic and transcriptomic analyses to define a subset of melanoma tumors with a specific transcriptomic signature (named IPRES) that are innately resistant to PD-1 checkpoint blockade. Ayers and colleagues[75] discovered an interferon-γ–related gene expression profile that is consistent with T-cell inflammation and that is an independent predictor of response to PD-1 blockade in 9 cancers. Other studies have found that the tumor mutation burden is a strong predictor of response to immunotherapy in both melanoma and NSCLC.[76,77] As such, although IHC-based techniques can be powerful on their own, combining these techniques with other assays, or further developing these techniques to become multiplexed and more quantitative, may help accelerate the discovery and validation of biomarkers.

## REFERENCES

1. Weber J, Mandala M, Del Vecchio M, et al. Adjuvant nivolumab versus ipilimumab in resected stage III or IV melanoma. N Engl J Med 2017;377:1824–35.

2. Walunas TL, Lenschow DJ, Bakker CY, et al. CTLA-4 can function as a negative regulator of T cell activation. Immunity 1994;1:405–13.

3. Krummel MF, Allison JP. CD28 and CTLA-4 have opposing effects on the response of T cells to stimulation. J Exp Med 1995;182:459–65.

4. Weber J, Thompson JA, Hamid O, et al. A randomized, double-blind, placebo-controlled, phase II study comparing the tolerability and efficacy of ipilimumab administered with or without prophylactic budesonide in patients with unresectable stage III or IV melanoma. Clin Cancer Res 2009;15:5591–8.

5. Wolchok JD, Neyns B, Linette G, et al. Ipilimumab monotherapy in patients with pretreated advanced melanoma: a randomised, double-blind, multicentre, phase 2, dose-ranging study. Lancet Oncol 2010;11:155–64.

6. O'Day SJ, Maio M, Chiarion-Sileni V, et al. Efficacy and safety of ipilimumab monotherapy in patients with pretreated advanced melanoma: a multicenter single-arm phase II study. Ann Oncol 2010;21:1712–7.

7. Eggermont AM, Chiarion-Sileni V, Grob JJ, et al. Prolonged survival in stage III melanoma with ipilimumab adjuvant therapy. N Engl J Med 2016;375:1845–55.

8. Hodi FS, O'Day SJ, McDermott DF, et al. Improved survival with ipilimumab in patients with metastatic melanoma. N Engl J Med 2010;363:711–23.

9. Topalian SL, Hodi FS, Brahmer JR, et al. Safety, activity, and immune correlates of anti-PD-1 antibody in cancer. N Engl J Med 2012;366:2443–54.

10. Patnaik A, Kang SP, Rasco D, et al. Phase I study of pembrolizumab (MK-3475; Anti-PD-1 monoclonal antibody) in patients with advanced solid tumors. Clin Cancer Res 2015;21:4286–93.

11. Brahmer JR, Tykodi SS, Chow LQ, et al. Safety and activity of anti-PD-L1 antibody in patients with advanced cancer. N Engl J Med 2012;366:2455–65.

12. Gong J, Chehrazi-Raffle A, Reddi S, et al. Development of PD-1 and PD-L1 inhibitors as a form of cancer immunotherapy: a comprehensive review of registration trials and future considerations. J Immunother Cancer 2018;6:8.

13. Wolchok JD, Kluger H, Callahan MK, et al. Nivolumab plus ipilimumab in advanced melanoma. N Engl J Med 2013;369:122–33.

14. Hellmann MD, Ciuleanu TE, Pluzanski A, et al. Nivolumab plus ipilimumab in lung cancer with a high tumor mutational burden. N Engl J Med 2018;378:2093–104.

15. Harris SJ, Brown J, Lopez J, et al. Immuno-oncology combinations: raising the tail of the survival curve. Cancer Biol Med 2016;13:171–93.

16. Postow MA, Callahan MK, Wolchok JD. Immune checkpoint blockade in cancer therapy. J Clin Oncol 2015;33:1974–82.

17. Freidlin B, Korn EL. Biomarker enrichment strategies: matching trial design to biomarker credentials. Nat Rev Clin Oncol 2014;11:81–90.

18. Nalejska E, Maczynska E, Lewandowska MA. Prognostic and predictive biomarkers: tools in personalized oncology. Mol Diagn Ther 2014;18:273–84.

19. Oldenhuis CN, Oosting SF, Gietema JA, et al. Prognostic versus predictive value of biomarkers in oncology. Eur J Cancer 2008;44:946–53.

20. Mabert K, Cojoc M, Peitzsch C, et al. Cancer biomarker discovery: current status and future perspectives. Int J Radiat Biol 2014;90:659–77.

21. Wolff AC, Hammond ME, Hicks DG, et al. Recommendations for human epidermal growth factor receptor 2 testing in breast cancer: American Society of Clinical Oncology/College of American Pathologists clinical practice guideline update. Arch Pathol Lab Med 2014;138:241–56.

22. Loupakis F, Pollina L, Stasi I, et al. PTEN expression and KRAS mutations on primary tumors and metastases in the prediction of benefit from cetuximab plus irinotecan for patients with metastatic colorectal cancer. J Clin Oncol 2009;27:2622–9.

23. Howat WJ, Lewis A, Jones P, et al. Antibody validation of immunohistochemistry for biomarker discovery: recommendations of a consortium of academic and pharmaceutical based histopathology researchers. Methods 2014;70:34–8.

24. Diamandis EP. The failure of protein cancer biomarkers to reach the clinic: why, and what can be done to address the problem? BMC Med 2012;10:87.

25. Oble DA, Loewe R, Yu P, et al. Focus on TILs: prognostic significance of tumor infiltrating lymphocytes in human melanoma. Cancer Immun 2009;9:3.

26. Weber CE, Kuo PC. The tumor microenvironment. Surg Oncol 2012;21:172–7.

27. Clemente CG, Mihm MC Jr, Bufalino R, et al. Prognostic value of tumor infiltrating lymphocytes in the vertical growth phase of primary cutaneous melanoma. Cancer 1996;77:1303–10.

28. Adams S, Gray RJ, Demaria S, et al. Prognostic value of tumor-infiltrating lymphocytes in triple-negative breast cancers from two phase III randomized adjuvant breast cancer trials: ECOG 2197 and ECOG 1199. J Clin Oncol 2014;32:2959–66.

29. Mihm MC Jr, Clemente CG, Cascinelli N. Tumor infiltrating lymphocytes in lymph node melanoma metastases: a histopathologic prognostic indicator and an expression of local immune response. Lab Invest 1996;74:43–7.

30. Hussein MR, Elsers DA, Fadel SA, et al. Immunohistological characterisation of tumour infiltrating lymphocytes in melanocytic skin lesions. J Clin Pathol 2006;59:316–24.

31. Loi S, Michiels S, Salgado R, et al. Tumor infiltrating lymphocytes are prognostic in triple negative breast cancer and predictive for trastuzumab benefit in early breast cancer: results from the FinHER trial. Ann Oncol 2014;25:1544–50.

32. Denkert C, Loibl S, Noske A, et al. Tumor-associated lymphocytes as an independent predictor of response to neoadjuvant chemotherapy in breast cancer. J Clin Oncol 2010;28:105–13.

33. Uryvaev A, Passhak M, Hershkovits D, et al. The role of tumor-infiltrating lymphocytes (TILs) as a predictive biomarker of response to anti-PD1 therapy in patients with metastatic non-small cell lung cancer or metastatic melanoma. Med Oncol 2018;35:25.

34. Sato E, Olson SH, Ahn J, et al. Intraepithelial CD8+ tumor-infiltrating lymphocytes and a high CD8+/regulatory T cell ratio are associated with favorable prognosis in ovarian cancer. Proc Natl Acad Sci U S A 2005;102:18538–43.

35. Mahmoud SM, Paish EC, Powe DG, et al. Tumor-infiltrating CD8+ lymphocytes predict clinical outcome in breast cancer. J Clin Oncol 2011;29:1949–55.

36. Liu H, Zhang T, Ye J, et al. Tumor-infiltrating lymphocytes predict response to chemotherapy in patients with advance non-small cell lung cancer. Cancer Immunol Immunother 2012;61:1849 56.

37. Liu S, Lachapelle J, Leung S, et al. CD8+ lymphocyte infiltration is an independent favorable prognostic indicator in basal-like breast cancer. Breast Cancer Res 2012;14:R48.

38. Erdag G, Schaefer JT, Smolkin ME, et al. Immunotype and immunohistologic characteristics of tumor-infiltrating immune cells are associated with clinical outcome in metastatic melanoma. Cancer Res 2012;72:1070–80.

39. Galon J, Costes A, Sanchez-Cabo F, et al. Type, density, and location of immune cells within human colorectal tumors predict clinical outcome. Science 2006;313:1960–4.

40. Piersma SJ, Jordanova ES, van Poelgeest MI, et al. High number of intraepithelial CD8+ tumor-infiltrating lymphocytes is associated with the absence of lymph node metastases in patients with large early-stage cervical cancer. Cancer Res 2007;67:354–61.

41. Tumeh PC, Harview CL, Yearley JH, et al. PD-1 blockade induces responses by inhibiting adaptive immune resistance. Nature 2014;515:568–71.

42. Lin J, Long J, Wan X, et al. Classification of gallbladder cancer by assessment of CD8(+) TIL and PD-L1 expression. BMC Cancer 2018;18:766.

43. Ameratunga M, Asadi K, Lin X, et al. PD-L1 and tumor infiltrating lymphocytes as prognostic markers in resected NSCLC. PLoS One 2016;11:e0153954.

44. Galon J, Mlecnik B, Bindea G, et al. Towards the introduction of the 'Immuno-score' in the classification of malignant tumours. J Pathol 2014;232:199–209.
45. Pages F, Mlecnik B, Marliot F, et al. International validation of the consensus Im-munoscore for the classification of colon cancer: a prognostic and accuracy study. Lancet 2018;391:2128–39.
46. Galon J, Fox BA, Bifulco CB, et al. Immunoscore and Immunoprofiling in cancer: an update from the melanoma and immunotherapy bridge 2015. J Transl Med 2016;14:273.
47. Ott PA, Hodi FS, Robert C. CTLA-4 and PD-1/PD-L1 blockade: new immunother-apeutic modalities with durable clinical benefit in melanoma patients. Clin Cancer Res 2013;19:5300–9.
48. Garon EB, Rizvi NA, Hui R, et al. Pembrolizumab for the treatment of non-small-cell lung cancer. N Engl J Med 2015;372:2018–28.
49. Khunger M, Hernandez AV, Pasupuleti V, et al. Programmed cell death 1 (PD-1) Ligand (PD-L1) expression in solid tumors as a predictive biomarker of benefit from PD-1/PD-L1 axis inhibitors: a systematic review and meta-analysis. JCO Pre-cis Oncol 2017;1:1–15.
50. Eggermont AMM, Blank CU, Mandala M, et al. Adjuvant pembrolizumab versus placebo in resected stage III melanoma. N Engl J Med 2018;378:1789–801.
51. Rimm DL, Han G, Taube JM, et al. A prospective, multi-institutional, pathologist-based assessment of 4 immunohistochemistry assays for PD-L1 expression in non-small cell lung cancer. JAMA Oncol 2017;3:1051–8.
52. Mathew M, Safyan RA, Shu CA. PD-L1 as a biomarker in NSCLC: challenges and future directions. Ann Transl Med 2017;5:375.
53. Hamid O, Schmidt H, Nissan A, et al. A prospective phase II trial exploring the association between tumor microenvironment biomarkers and clinical activity of ipilimumab in advanced melanoma. J Transl Med 2011;9:204.
54. Quezada SA, Peggs KS, Curran MA, et al. CTLA4 blockade and GM-CSF com-bination immunotherapy alters the intratumor balance of effector and regulatory T cells. J Clin Invest 2006;116:1935–45.
55. Hodi FS, Butler M, Oble DA, et al. Immunologic and clinical effects of antibody blockade of cytotoxic T lymphocyte-associated antigen 4 in previously vacci-nated cancer patients. Proc Natl Acad Sci U S A 2008;105:3005–10.
56. Berman DM, Wolchok J, Weber J, et al. Association of peripheral blood absolute lymphocyte count (ALC) and clinical activity in patients (PTS) with advanced mel-anoma treated with ipilimumab. J Clin Oncol 2009;27:3020.
57. Cha E, Klinger M, Hou Y, et al. Improved survival with T cell clonotype stability af-ter anti-CTLA-4 treatment in cancer patients. Sci Transl Med 2014;6:238ra70.
58. Postow MA, Manuel M, Wong P, et al. Peripheral T cell receptor diversity is asso-ciated with clinical outcomes following ipilimumab treatment in metastatic mela-noma. J Immunother Cancer 2015;3:23.
59. Manson G, Norwood J, Marabelle A, et al. Biomarkers associated with checkpoint inhibitors. Ann Oncol 2016;27:1199–206.
60. McCabe A, Dolled-Filhart M, Camp RL, et al. Automated quantitative analysis (AQUA) of in situ protein expression, antibody concentration, and prognosis. J Natl Cancer Inst 2005;97:1808–15.
61. O'Hurley G, Sjostedt E, Rahman A, et al. Garbage in, garbage out: a critical eval-uation of strategies used for validation of immunohistochemical biomarkers. Mol Oncol 2014;8:783–98.
62. Saper CB. A guide to the perplexed on the specificity of antibodies. J Histochem Cytochem 2009;57:1–5.

63. Bordeaux J, Welsh A, Agarwal S, et al. Antibody validation. Biotechniques 2010; 48:197–209.
64. Williams JH, Mepham BL, Wright DH. Tissue preparation for immunocytochemistry. J Clin Pathol 1997;50:422–8.
65. Joshi AS, Sharangpani GM, Porter K, et al. Semi-automated imaging system to quantitate Her-2/neu membrane receptor immunoreactivity in human breast cancer. Cytometry A 2007;71:273–85.
66. Gartrell RD, Marks DK, Hart TD, et al. Quantitative analysis of immune infiltrates in primary melanoma. Cancer Immunol Res 2018;6:481–93.
67. Johnson DB, Bordeaux JM, Kim JY, et al. Quantitative spatial profiling of PD-1/PD-L1 interaction and HLA-DR/IDO-1 Predicts improved outcomes of anti-PD-1 therapies in metastatic melanoma. Clin Cancer Res 2018;24:5250–60.
68. Carstens JL, Correa de Sampaio P, Yang D, et al. Spatial computation of intratumoral T cells correlates with survival of patients with pancreatic cancer. Nat Commun 2017;8:15095.
69. Ali HR, Dariush A, Provenzano E, et al. Computational pathology of pre-treatment biopsies identifies lymphocyte density as a predictor of response to neoadjuvant chemotherapy in breast cancer. Breast Cancer Res 2016;18:21.
70. Feng Z, Bethmann D, Kappler M, et al. Multiparametric immune profiling in HPV-oral squamous cell cancer. JCI Insight 2017;2 [pii:93652].
71. Landers KA, Burger MJ, Tebay MA, et al. Use of multiple biomarkers for a molecular diagnosis of prostate cancer. Int J Cancer 2005;114:950–6.
72. Wang K, Huang C, Nice EC. Proteomics, genomics and transcriptomics: their emerging roles in the discovery and validation of colorectal cancer biomarkers. Expert Rev Proteomics 2014;11:179–205.
73. Dijkstra KK, Voabil P, Schumacher TN, et al. Genomics- and transcriptomics-based patient selection for cancer treatment with immune checkpoint inhibitors: a review. JAMA Oncol 2016;2:1490–5.
74. Hugo W, Zaretsky JM, Sun L, et al. Genomic and transcriptomic features of response to anti-PD-1 therapy in metastatic melanoma. Cell 2016;165:35–44.
75. Ayers M, Lunceford J, Nebozhyn M, et al. IFN-gamma-related mRNA profile predicts clinical response to PD-1 blockade. J Clin Invest 2017;127:2930–40.
76. Van Allen EM, Miao D, Schilling B, et al. Genomic correlates of response to CTLA-4 blockade in metastatic melanoma. Science 2015;350:207–11.
77. Rizvi NA, Hellmann MD, Snyder A, et al. Cancer immunology. Mutational landscape determines sensitivity to PD-1 blockade in non-small cell lung cancer. Science 2015;348:124–8.

# Special Articles

# Immunotherapy for Head and Neck Cancer

Felix Sim, MBBS, BDS, FRACDS(OMS)[a,b,c], Rom Leidner, MD[d],
Richard Bryan Bell, MD, DDS[d,e],*

## KEYWORDS

- Head and neck cancer • Squamous cell carcinoma • Immunotherapy
- Checkpoint inhibitor • Oncolytic virus • Adoptive T-cell transfer

## KEY POINTS

- Cancer immunotherapy relies on the recognition of tumor cells as a foreign antigen, which then becomes the target of attack of an activated immune system.
- Immunotherapy is thought to have a distinct advantage over cytotoxic chemotherapy and targeted therapy due to the potential durable response from memory T cells.
- Two anti–PD-1 antibodies, nivolumab and pembrolizumab, have shown efficacy in clinical trials for recurrent metastatic HNSCC and were approved by the US Food and Drug Administration for use in the second-line setting in 2016.
- Head and neck squamous cell carcinomas (HNSCC) are known for their immune-suppressive character and early single modality immunotherapy treatments have only yielded a modest response rate when compared with melanoma.
- The challenge for clinicians is to understand how and in which clinical setting to use these agents to provide greatest clinical benefit for patients.

## INTRODUCTION

Advances in immunotherapy have transformed the practice of oncology. Immunotherapy for treatment of cancer relies on the principle that tumors are recognized as

This article originally appeared in *Oral and Maxillofacial Surgery Clinics of North America*, Volume 31, Issue 1, February 2019.
Disclosure Statement: The authors have nothing to disclose.
[a] Department of Oral and Maxillofacial Surgery, The Royal Melbourne Hospital, 300 Grattan Street, Parkville, Victoria 3050, Australia; [b] Department of Oral and Maxillofacial Surgery, Monash Health, 823 Centre Road, Bentleigh East, Victoria 3165, Australia; [c] Oral and Maxillofacial Surgery Unit, Barwon Health, Ryrie Street & Bellerine Street, Geelong, Victoria 3220, Australia; [d] Earle A. Chiles Research Institute, Robert W. Franz Cancer Center, Providence Portland Medical Center, Providence Cancer Institute, 4805 Northeast Glisan Street, Suite 2N35, Portland, OR 97213, USA; [e] Head and Neck Institute, 1849 NW Kearney, Suite 300, Portland, Oregon 97209, USA
* Corresponding author. Providence Portland Medical Center, 4805 Northeast Glisan Street, Suite 6N50, Portland, OR 97213.
*E-mail address:* richard.bell@providence.org

Hematol Oncol Clin N Am 33 (2019) 301–321
https://doi.org/10.1016/j.hoc.2018.12.006
0889-8588/19/© 2018 Elsevier Inc. All rights reserved.

foreign by the host immune cells and can be effectively destroyed by an activated immune system. Through a better understanding of the various mechanisms of control of immunity, checkpoint inhibitors, such as anticytotoxic T-lymphocyte–associated protein 4 (anti–CTLA-4) and anti-programmed cell death protein-1 (anti–PD-1) have resulted in durable responses and improved survival in patients with advanced cancer. Other strategies currently under exploration include adoptive cell transfer with tumor-infiltrating lymphocytes (TILs) or engineered antigen receptor T cells.

Patients with head and neck squamous cell carcinomas (HNSCCs) have a relatively poor prognosis, which despite 5 decades of advancements in surgery, radiation therapy, and chemotherapy, has not significantly improved. Treatment for recurrent/metastatic (R/M) HNSCC is especially challenging, regardless of human papilloma virus (HPV) status, with few effective treatment options. HPV-negative HNSCC is associated with a local-regional relapse rate of 19% to 35% and a distant metastatic rate of 14% to 22% following standard of care, compared with rates of 9% to 18% and 5% to 12%, respectively, for HPV-positive HNSCC.[1–3] The median overall survival (OS) for patients with recurrent metastatic disease is 10 to 13 months in the setting of first-line chemotherapy and 6 months in the second-line setting. The current standard of care is platinum-based doublet chemotherapy with or without cetuximab. Until recently, second-line standard of care options included only cetuximab, methotrexate, and taxanes, all of which were associated with significant side effects and a low response rate of 10% to 13%. Regression of HNSCC from treatment with chemotherapy alone is most often transient, does not significantly increase longevity, and fails to prevent virtually all patients from succumbing to malignancy.

In 2016, 2 anti-PD1 antibodies, nivolumab and pembrolizumab, were shown to improve OS in patients with recurrent, metastatic HNSCC and were approved by the US Food and Drug Administration (FDA) for use in the second-line setting.[4,5] The result has been a new standard of care for platinum-resistant, R/M HNSCC. Compared with standard cytotoxic chemotherapy, immunotherapy improves OS with durable responses to therapy, generating the so-called "tail on the (Kaplan-Meier) curve" (**Fig. 1**). Despite this encouraging progress, response rates to PD-1/PD-L1 inhibitors in HNSCC range from 13% to 20%, whereas survival is improved in just 1 of 10 patients treated. An enormous effort is under way to develop novel therapeutic approaches aimed toward stimulating immunity in cancer. This article reviews the immunotherapies currently in clinical trials for patients with HNSCC and discusses ongoing efforts to enhance response rates and integrate immunotherapy into the definitive-treatment setting.

## IMMUNOSURVEILLANCE AND IMMUNOEDITING OF CANCER

Richmond Prehn and Joan Main[6] demonstrated the immunologic specificity of tumors by showing that tumors induced by chemical carcinogens in mice stimulate tumor-specific responses that reject those same tumors on subsequent inoculation, whereas spontaneous-arising tumors were not rejected. Burnet[7] later confirmed this observation and coined the term "immunosurveillance," suggesting that tumor cells express antigens different from normal cells, and therefore, can be identified as "nonself" by the circulating lymphocytes for clearance.

Immunosurveillance of cancer is a coordinated process involving both the innate and adaptive immune system. Innate immunity refers to the part of the immune system that provides antigen-nonspecific, first-line protection. Effectors of innate immunity include natural killer (NK) cells, neutrophils, macrophages, dendritic cells (DCs), and monocytes that attack and ingest pathogens. Innate immunity is nonspecific and lacks efficacy after repeated exposures to the same antigenic challenge.

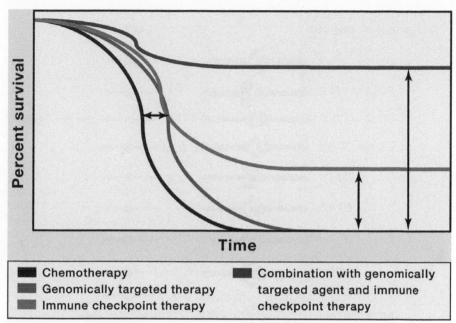

**Chemotherapy**
**Genomically targeted therapy**
**Immune checkpoint therapy**

**Combination with genomically
targeted agent and immune
checkpoint therapy**

**Fig. 1.** The promise of immunotherapy: the Kaplan-Meier curve tail. Previously, cancer thera-pies, such genomically targeted therapies or chemotherapy, would extend progression-free in-tervals for most patients with metastatic cancer, but OS was not improved. Virtually all patients still died, as indicated by the horizontal change in the survival curve. With immune checkpoint therapy, not as many patients respond to treatment, but a percentage of those who do respond will receive lasting benefit, as evidenced by the vertical change in the OS curves (ie, the "tail on the curve"). It is postulated that the combination of checkpoint inhibitors with other immunotherapies and genomically targeted agents will further improve OS in the future. (*From* Sharma P, Allison JP. Immune checkpoint targeting in cancer therapy: toward combination strategies with curative potential. Cell 2015;161(2):211; with permission.)

The adaptive immune system is triggered by the innate immune response, on the other hand, may have a durable effect. DCs and antigen-presenting cells (APCs) ingest and present these tumor antigens bound to major histocompatibility complex (MHC) class I or MHC class II signaling through the T-cell receptor, the first signal in T-cell proliferation. This process usually occurs in the regional lymph nodes. The activation and differentiation of these tumor-specific T cells requires 2 additional signals, the second termed costimulation and the third signal consisting of a variety of cytokines, such as interleukin (IL)-12 or type 1 interferon (IFN), to avoid T-cell tolerance or death. Once activated, effector T cells can be modulated by antibodies targeting positive costimulatory signals, via receptors such as OX-40 or 4-1BB, or negative co-inhibitory signals, such as CTLA-4 or PD-1, which causes apoptosis of T cells on bind-ing to their cogent receptor (**Fig. 2**).

Identifying tumor antigen-specific T cells from patients with cancer has important implications for immunotherapy diagnostics and therapeutics. Recently, Duhen and colleagues[8] showed that CD103+ CD39+ tumor-infiltrating CD8 TILs are enriched for tumor-reactive cells both in primary and metastatic tumors across 6 different ma-lignancies. CD103 + CD39 + CD8 TILs also efficiently kill autologous tumor cells in an MHC class I–dependent manner. Correlating this clinically, patients with HNSCC with higher frequencies of CD103 + CD39 + CD8 TILs had better OS. The ability to detect

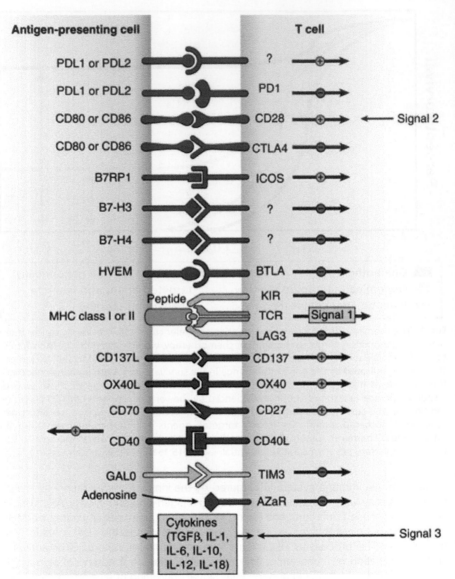

**Fig. 2.** Regulation of T-cell response. T-cell activation is mediated by peptide-MHC molecule complexes that are recognized by the TCR and modulated through various ligand–receptor interactions between T cells and APCs. In the presence of a "maturation signal," such as Toll-like receptor ligands, APCs can migrate to the regional lymph nodes and process the TAA. Once in the draining lymph node, tumor antigens presented via MHC molecules on APC's initiate activation and differentiation of tumor-specific T cells. Activation requires a second signal, termed costimulation, via the (B7) CD80/86:CD28 receptor complex. Signal 2 generally consists of pairs of costimulatory-inhibitory receptors that bind the same ligand or ligands, such as CD28 and CTLA4 and display distinct kinetics of expression with the costimulatory receptor expressed on naive and resting T cells. However, the inhibitory receptor is commonly upregulated after T-cell activation. The B7 family of membrane-bound ligands are particularly important in that they bind to both costimulatory and inhibitory receptors. TNF family members, on the other hand, bind to cognate TNF receptor family

tumor-reactive CD8 TILs will help define mechanisms of existing immunotherapy treatments, and may lead to more effective adoptive T-cell cancer therapies.

Further elaboration of immunosurveillance led to the concept of "immunoediting". Immunoediting is a dynamic evolutionary process whereby immune surveillance of cancers provides selective pressure on tumor cells and negatively selects for cells that can evade the immune system.[9] The end result is successful tumor progression occurring only after the tumor has discovered a means by which it can evade the immune system. Cancer immunoediting consists of 3 potential phases: elimination, equilibrium, and escape. In the elimination phase, the innate and adaptive immune response destroys developing malignancies before they become clinically apparent. Ideally, all tumor cells are eliminated in this phase and the host remains free of cancer. However, some tumor cells may remain and enter the equilibrium phase, in which tumor progression is kept in check by immunologic mechanisms, and subclinical disease remains stable. Equilibrium is a function of adaptive immunity only. Over time, however, some tumors develop "escape mechanisms," such that cancer cells are no longer recognized by the adaptive immune response due to antigen loss or defects in the antigen-processing machinery, insensitivity to immune effector mechanisms, or the induction of immunosuppressive mechanisms within the tumor microenvironment (TME), such as expression of PD-L1, an inhibitory receptor on the tumor surface (**Fig. 3**).

## MECHANISMS OF IMMUNE ESCAPE IN HEAD AND NECK SQUAMOUS CELL CARCINOMA

Analysis of the TME in patients with a variety of solid tumors has shown 2 major subsets of tumors with distinct mechanisms of resistance to immune-mediated destruction. Tumors with an inflamed phenotype appeared to have high recruitment of T cells, triggered by the presence of immune signals and chemokines. Immunohistochemical staining confirmed the abundance of CD8+ cytotoxic T cells, macrophages, and B cells in these tumors. In these tumor types, immune resistance occurs after T-cell migration into the TME, implying the inhibitory influence of immune signaling pathway. In noninflamed tumors, TME lack T cells and other effectors of innate immunity, such as chemokines. Immune escape is attributed to poor effector T-cell trafficking, as required signaling pathways are absent.[10]

The authors have shown in both preclinical models and human subjects with HNSCC that the curative potential of surgery is significantly affected by the interactions between the effector (CD4+ and CD8+ T cells) and suppressive elements (regulatory T cells [T-regs] and PD-L1+ tumor cells) of the immune infiltrate in the TME.[11] Using sophisticated multiplex immunohistochemical staining (mIHC) and multispectral

---

molecules and deliver primarily costimulatory signals. In addition to antigen (Ag) presentation and costimulation, a third signal consisting of a variety of cytokines, such as IL-12 or Type I IFN, is required to avoid T-cell tolerance or death. Antigen presentation via MHC is insufficient without all 3 signals and will result in T-cell tolerance (anergy). Communication between T cells and APCs is bidirectional. In some cases, this occurs when ligands themselves signal to the APC. In other cases, activated T cells upregulate ligands, such as CD40L, that engage cognate receptors on APCs. A2aR, adenosine A2a receptor; B7RP1, B7-related protein 1; BTLA, B and T lymphocyte attenuator; GAL9, galectin 9; HVEM, herpesvirus entry mediator; ICOS, inducible T-cell costimulator; LAG3, lymphocyte activation gene 3; PD1, programmed cell death protein 1; PDL, PD1 ligand; TIM3, T-cell membrane protein 3. (*Adapted from* Pardoll D. The blockade of immune checkpoints in cancer immunotherapy. Nat Rev Cancer 2012;12(4):254; with permission.)

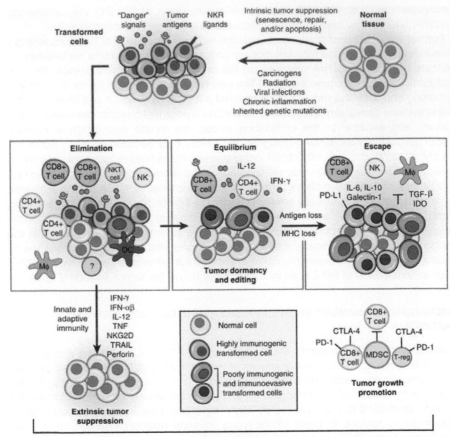

**Fig. 3.** The cancer immunoediting concept. Cancer immunoediting consists of 3 potential phases: elimination, equilibrium, and escape. In the elimination phase, the innate and adaptive immune systems destroy developing malignancies before they become clinically apparent. Ideally, all tumor cells are eliminated in this phase and the host remains free of cancer, in which case the process is complete. However, if tumor cells are allowed to remain, the host then enters the equilibrium phase, in which tumor progression is kept in check by immunologic mechanisms and subclinical disease remains stable. Equilibrium is a function of adaptive immunity only. It is possible that the cancer immunoediting process may prevent clinical progression for the lifetime of the host and is the terminal process. Over time, however, some tumors develop "escape mechanisms," such that cancer cells are no longer recognized by the adaptive immune system due to antigen loss or defects in antigen-processing machinery, insensitivity to immune effector mechanisms, or the induction of immunosuppressive mechanisms within the TME, such as PD-L1. These cancer cells then proliferate, causing clinically significant disease, with the ability to metastasize and kill the host. NKT, natural killer T-cell. (*Adapted from* Schreiber RD, Old LJ, Smyth MJ. Cancer immunoediting: integrating immunity's roles in cancer suppression and promotion. Science 2011;331:1567; with permission.)

imaging techniques to enumerate immune cell types and cartographic coordinates of each cell in formalin-fixed paraffin-embedded tissue, we developed a cumulative suppressive index (CSI), which is a highly significant prognostic biomarker ($P<.0005$) for OS in patients with HPV-negative (HPV−) HNSCC (**Fig. 4**). Understanding the function

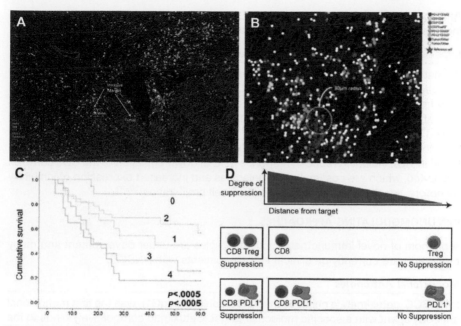

**Fig. 4.** CSI is a highly significant prognostic biomarker for patients with surgically treated HNSCC. (*A*) mIHC with simultaneous stain for 7 Ag, focusing on highest density of immune cell infiltrate at the stroma and the invasive margin (IM). (*B*) CSI scoring system combines the evaluation of FoxP3+ and PD-L1+ within 30 μm of CD8+ T cells at both the stromal and tumor side of the IM. (*C*) Kaplan-Meier curve of a cohort of 119 surgically treated patients with HPV-HNSCC demonstrating a highly significant stepwise reduction of OS based on an increasing CSI, with 0 representing the lowest and 4 representing the most suppression relative to CD8+ T cells. (*D*) Immunosuppression as it relates to spacial relationships of suppressor to effector elements in the TME.

of these CD8 T-cell subsets within tumors and how they evolve and respond to immunotherapy will increase our knowledge of what cells are important for tumor rejection in humans and what antigens they are responding to.

HNSCC cancer cells use several strategies to evade immune recognition and destruction for ongoing tumor proliferation.

## *Upregulation of Regulatory T Cells in the Tumor Microenvironment*

One of the major cellular components within the TME is T-regs, which are defined by coexpression of CD4, FoxP3, and CD25 on its cell membrane. HNSCC-derived suppressive factors can condition T cells and myeloid cells to adopt suppressive features, converting them to T-regs and myeloid-derived suppressor cells (MDSCs).[12] T-regs in TME express immune checkpoint receptors such as CTLA-4 and PD-1, as well as immunosuppressive molecules such as CD-39 and transforming growth factor (TGF)-β1. High numbers of T-regs in TILs have correlated with poor survival in a number of reports.[13–15]

## *Disruption of Antigen-Presenting Mechanism*

The upregulation of MDSCs in TME produce inflammatory mediators such as IL-1, IL-6, inducible nitric oxide synthase (iNOS), and reactive oxygen species, which impair

APC maturation.[12] Baseline levels of MDSCs increase with age and may contribute to increased tumor frequency and growth rate with increased age.[16]

### Impaired Function of Immune Effector Cells

As stated previously, activation of cytotoxic T cells relies on the balance of inhibitory and stimulatory signaling mediated by DCs and T-helper cells (Th cells). In peripheral blood of patients with HNSCC, although cytotoxic T cells are identified in lower concentrations, effector memory T cells are found in a higher percentage, suggesting initial T-cell recognition of tumor antigen.[17,18] However, HNSCC induces T-cell anergy in both peripheral T lymphocytes and TILs.[10] Intrinsic molecular defects have been found in TILs, including reduced response to IL-2, downregulation of the CD3 complex and OX40, which are costimulatory molecules and increased expression of inhibitory receptors, such as PD-1 and CTLA-4 for T-cell proliferation.[19–21]

## IMMUNOMODULATING APPROACHES

A plethora of novel immunotherapeutic strategies are under development and many treatments are currently on clinical trials for patients with HNSCC.

### Monoclonal Antibodies

In HNSCC, cetuximab, a chimeric immunoglobulin G1 (IgG1), was the first monoclonal antibody agent with a specific molecular target. Cetuximab competitively binds to the epidermal growth factor receptor (EGFR), preventing activation of the receptor by endogenous ligands. EGFR is overexpressed in 80% to 90% of cases of HNSCC, enabling tumor cell proliferation, invasion, angiogenesis, and tumor survival. Overexpression of EGFR has been associated with poor survival and prognosis.[22] Cetuximab is approved by the FDA for use in combination with radiation in locally advanced HNSCC and with chemotherapy in recurrent, metastatic disease.[23,24] Cetuximab induces an antibody-dependent cell-mediated cytotoxicity (ADCC), by activating FCγRIIIa, an Fc receptor on the surface of NK cells, which mediates ADCC and triggers the release of IFNγ in response to antibody-coated target cells. Cetuximab also stimulates cytotoxic T-cell antitumor response through cross-priming of DCs and NKs.[25]

### Immune Checkpoint Inhibitors

The investigation of checkpoint blockade antibodies is at the forefront of immunotherapy. Blocking these immune checkpoints with antibodies results in restoration of T-cell function and an enhanced antitumor response in some patients. Although most of the trials to date have investigated anti–CTLA-4, anti–PD-1, and anti–PD-L1, other novel checkpoint blockade inhibitors are being tested in both preclinical and clinical settings for HNSCC.

#### Anti–cytotoxic T-lymphocyte–associated protein-4

CTLA-4 is a CD28 homologue expressed on the surface of T lymphocytes.[26] CTLA-4 is expressed transiently on the surface of early activated CD8 T cells and constitutively on T-regs.[27] The mechanism of inhibition of CD8+ T cells by CTLA-4 involves engagement of costimulatory molecules CD80 and CD86 to CTLA-4 on CD8 T cells, resulting in dephosphorylation of T-cell receptor (TCR) signaling proteins, such as CD3, and leading to T-cell anergy. In addition, CTLA-4 has higher affinity for CD80/CD86 than CD28, effectively reducing the availability of signal 2 required for activation of CD8 T cells. Antibodies that block CTLA-4 receptors result in significantly increased CD8 T-cell activation and proliferation in preclinical models.[28,29] Ipilimumab (anti–CTLA-

4) was approved for the treatment of metastatic melanoma in 2011 based on a randomized phase III study demonstrating superior efficacy when compared with gp100 vaccine alone.[30] The efficacy and safety of anti–CTLA-4 in head and neck cancer is currently under investigation in a phase Ib trial in combination with cetuximab and intensity-modulated radiation therapy for patients with previously untreated stage III-IVB head and neck cancer (NCT01935921).

*Anti–programmed cell death protein-1*

PD-1 is also an inhibitory receptor expressed on T-cell activation.[31] Similar to CTLA-4, binding of PD-1 to its ligand PD-L1 induces dephosphorylation of CD3, resulting in T-cell suppresion.[17] When PD-1 binding to PD-L1 is inhibited by an anti–PD-1 agent, restoration of CD8 T-cell function augmented antitumor activity in numerous preclinical models[18,32–34] and significantly improved survival in patients with melanoma, renal cell carcinoma, and non–small-cell lung carcinoma.[35–37] In melanoma, rates of response and OS have been further increased by anti–PD-1 in combination with an anti–CTLA-4.[35,38]

The recent results of 2 trials of PD-1 checkpoint inhibition for patients with HNSCC have paved the way to a new standard of care. A phase III trial, Checkmate 141, compared the anti–PD-1 antibody nivolumab versus standard of care for metastatic HNSCC and was halted early when survival endpoints were met.[5] The interim results demonstrated improved survival in patients with HNSCC who progressed within 6 months of platinum therapy as part of first-line treatment for recurrent metastatic disease. Nivolumab reduced the risk of death by 30% compared with investigator's choice of standard chemotherapy and doubled the 1-year OS from 16.6% in the control arm to 36% in the nivolumab arm. Median survival was 7.5 months for nivolumab and 5.1 months for patients assigned to investigator's choice of chemotherapy.

Another anti–PD-1 antibody, pembrolizumab, was investigated by Seiwert and colleagues[4] in the phase I trial KEYNOTE-012 for patients with recurrent metastatic HNSCC. The overall response rate was 18% (25% in HPV-positive patients and 14% in HPV-negative patients). These encouraging results led to approval by the FDA in 2016 for pembrolizumab and nivolumab in second-line treatment of metastatic HNSCC.[39] It is worth noting that a recent follow-up phase III trial of pembrolizumab versus standard chemotherapy with methotrexate, docetaxel or cetuximab, and pembrolizumab did not meet the primary endpoint of OS. Patients receiving pembrolizumab had an overall 19% improvement in OS that did not meet the prespecified difference for statistical significance. Nonetheless, pembrolizumab was less toxic compared with the investigator's choice of chemotherapy, an important consideration in treatment of patients with a poor prognosis for recurrent metastatic platinum-refractory HNSCC.[40]

Recently, 2 phase I trials were opened for accrual to investigate nivolumab (NCT02488759) and pembrolizumab (NCT02296684) before surgery for patients with HNSCC. These trials are recruiting patients with both HPV-positive and HPV-negative tumors to determine the effects of PD-1 blockade in the TME of HNSCC. Their results will set the stage to investigate the addition of anti–PD-1 to adjuvant therapy for patients with locoregionally advanced disease.

*Anti–programmed cell death protein-L1*

The binding of PD-1 and its cell-surface ligand PD-L1 results in T-cell inhibition.[41] PD-L1 is expressed in a multitude of tissues, including muscles and nerves. Of relevance for cancer immunotherapy, PD-L1 can be expressed on the surface of tumor cells, tumor-associated macrophages, and T lymphocytes, which can subsequently inhibit

PD-1–positive T cells.[42] The expression of PD-L1 can be induced by cytokines, such as IFNs or by autonomous aberrations in EGFR signaling pathways.[43–45] To date, there are 3 anti–PD-L1 agents that have been approved by the FDA for urothelial carcinoma, atezolizumab, durvalumab, and avelumab. In HNSCC, anti–PD-L1 agents are under investigation in multiple phase I and II clinical trials in combination with other agents.

### Other checkpoint blockades

A number of immune checkpoint inhibitors have been developed and several are currently under investigation either in the preclinical setting or in clinical trials for the treatment of patients with cancer. Two examples of agents that have moved into the clinical trial setting are anti-lymphocyte activation gene 3 (anti–LAG-3), which targets an inhibitory receptor on the surface of T cells, and anti–killer cell immunoglobulin-like receptor (KIR), which acts to reverse NK cell inhibition, an important source of impaired innate immunity.

Trials involving anti–LAG-3 alone and in combination with anti–PD-1 are ongoing in the treatment of hematologic and advanced solid malignancies, including HNSCC, and the results are eagerly awaited. Although these combinations are hoped to improve response rates in treatment of solid tumors, one highly anticipated phase I/II trial that targeted both innate (lirilumab, anti-KIR) and adaptive (nivolumab, anti–PD-1) immunity failed to meet clinical endpoints. The interim analysis in a cohort of 29 patients with advanced platinum-refractory HNSCC showed 3 patients with a complete response (10.3%) and 4 patients with a partial response (13.8%), along with a reduction in tumor size of more than 80% and a 12-month OS rate of 60% with lirilumab plus nivolumab (NCT01714739). A recent update of this trial in an expanded cohort showed no clear evidence of benefit for patients treated with lirilumab combined with nivolumab compared with nivolumab alone, thus casting doubt on the possibility of FDA approval for lirilumab.[46]

### Costimulatory Agonists

Costimulatory molecules, such as anti-OX40 and anti-4-1BB, cause T-cell proliferation, memory, cytotoxic effector function, and cytokine production. An agonist antibody that targets the tumor necrosis factor receptor (TNFR) family member, 4-1BB, has shown therapeutic responses in preclinical mouse models.[47] A similar agonist antibody to OX40 was described in 2000 by Weinberg and colleagues,[29] who demonstrated therapeutic effects and enhanced T-cell function in numerous mouse models.

### Anti-OX40

OX40 is a member of the TNFR superfamily and is present on the surface of T cells, in particular CD4 T cells and T-regs.[48,49] Activation of OX40 through an agonist antibody, either directly or indirectly, increases CD4 and CD8 T-cell priming and proliferation. Inhibiting the function of CD8 T cells appears to be hindered partly through the disruption of FOXP3 expression and inhibitory cytokine release.[50] The result may tip the effector-to-suppressor balance in the TME as an explanation for the significant antitumor efficacy in many immunogenic preclinical models.[51] Clinically, MEDI6469, an agonist antibody to OX40, has demonstrated safety in a phase I trial,[52] and the antibody is currently under investigation as a single agent in the neoadjuvant setting for the treatment of patients with HNSCC (NCT02274155).

### 4-1BB

4-1BB is another member of the TNFR superfamily stably expressed on activated T cells and NK cells.[53] Activation by 4-1BB ligand or by an agonist antibody on CD8

T cells results in increased proliferation, cytokine production, and survival. 4-1BB activation also has a profound impact on the humoral immune system and CD4 T cells.[54] There are several ongoing phase I/II trials evaluating 4-1BB agonists (Urelumab, Utomilumab) in combination with cetuximab (NCT02110082), Nivolumab (NCT02253992), or other costimulatory agents (NCT02315066) in HNSCC.[55]

## Adoptive T-Cell Transfer

Adoptive T-cell transfer (ACT) involves harvesting T cells from autologous tumor resection specimen or biopsy, expanding them ex vivo with IL-2, testing for tumor specificity, and then rapidly expanding them for reinfusion into a nonmyeloablative lymphodepleted patient. Initial work on ACT originated from successful treatment of metastatic melanoma with adoptive transfers of TILs. Investigators from the National Cancer Institute reported the results of ACT in 93 patients with metastatic melanoma who received TILs after a lymphodepleting regimen plus IL-2 (aldesleukin) administration, with or without total body irradiation.[56] The overall response rate using the Response Evaluation Criteria in Solid Tumors in 93 patients was 56%. Of the 52 responding patients in this trial, 42 had disease that was refractory to aldesleukin therapy and 22 had disease that was refractory to prior aldesleukin plus chemotherapy. This TIL therapy shows promise as an effective treatment for chemotherapy-refractory metastatic melanoma and led to investigation in other malignancies.

ACT has been used in HNSCC with one center reporting a remarkable Response Rate of 43% in the 7 patients studied.[57] The significant barrier to ACT is the ability to culture and expand tumor-specific T cells from the patients' autologous tumors. In renal, breast, and colon cancer, the recovery rate is extremely low (0%–20%).[58] In HNSCC, however, the success rate in obtaining tumor-specific T cells from autologous tumors is approximately 60%.[59] An effort to commercialize ACT for the treatment of solid tumors has recently begun. Iovance (San Carlos, CA), a biotechnology company, is sponsoring an ongoing trial in patients with HNSCC, which involves central tissue processing and TIL expansion at numerous sites across the United States (NCT03083873).[60]

## Vaccines

Cancer vaccines aim to generate tumor regression through activation of the adaptive immune system by the processing and presentation of tumor-specific antigens for T-cell recognition. It is currently hypothesized that a preexisting antitumor T-cell response is critical for the therapeutic effects of checkpoint blockade, especially for anti–PD-1. For patients lacking this preexisting tumor-specific immune response, priming a new antitumor response through vaccines might provide substantial benefit to therapy involving checkpoint blockade or immune system agonists. There are 5 main types of vaccines, discussed in the following sections.

### Peptide and whole-protein vaccine
Peptide or whole-protein vaccines are engineered to mimic tumor-associated antigen (TAA). These molecules then bind via MHC to the surface of APCs and are directly presented to T cells.

### Whole-cell vaccine
Whole-cell vaccines are prepared using irradiated whole tumor cells and are frequently delivered with an adjuvant, such as granulocyte-macrophase colony-stimulating factor (GM-CSF). Whole-cell vaccine has an advantage over peptide vaccine in containing a richer antigenic source.

### Autophagosome-based vaccines

Autophagy is a process by which cells recycle cellular components through autophagolysosomal fusion. Tumor autophagy is necessary for tumor-specific T-cell priming through induction of cross-presentation of tumor antigens by DCs. Tumor-derived autophagosomes contain short-lived proteins and defective ribosomal products. These 2 proteins degrade rapidly in whole-cell vaccine, but are captured and enriched in autophagosome-based vaccines. Short-lived proteins and defective ribosomal product (Dribble) vaccines have been shown to be more effective than the laboratory's gold standard GM-CSF gene-modified (GVAX) tumor vaccine.[61] This strategy of using tumor-derived autophagosome vaccines to share tumor antigens is under investigation by the authors for the treatment of HNSCC and oral dysplasia.

### Oncolytic virus vaccine

Oncolytic viruses specifically target tumor cells and function through a combination of tumor cell lysis and stimulation of innate and adaptive immunity by presenting viral and tumor antigens. Cellular entry of virus occurs through virus-specific receptor-mediated mechanisms. An example of this is Cavatak, a coxsackievirus developed by Viralytics (Sydney, Australia), which seeks out and attaches itself to a protein that is highly expressed on the surface of many cancer cells, intercellular adhesion molecule-1 (ICAM-1). Because ICAM-1 is expressed in HNSCC,[62] a phase 1 clinical trial studying Cavatak with pembrolizumab has been designed and is currently in its final stages of preparation before opening for recruitment. In a similar concept, a multicenter trial combining a modified herpes simplex virus, talimogene laherparepvec (T-VEC) with pembrolizumab is currently recruiting patients with recurrent metastatic HNSCC (NCT02626000). Another example, T-VEC, the only oncolytic virus with current FDA approval, has use in the treatment of melanoma.

## RADIOTHERAPY AND IMMUNOTHERAPY

Radiation therapy (RT) is often used as an adjuvant treatment following surgery for patients with HNSCC. Conventional RT approaches consist of either definitive chemoradiotherapy to 70 Gy delivered over 6 to 7 weeks, or primary surgery followed by risk-adapted radiotherapy alone delivered over 6 weeks or chemoradiation with high-dose cisplatin 100 mg/m$^2$ for 3 cycles. Concurrent chemoradiation as treatment for patients with HNSCC over 6 to 7 weeks is highly toxic and generally considered one of the most intensive treatment regimens in all of oncology.

Hypofractionated radiation may have both clinical and biologic advantage over standard fractionation, in reducing toxicity and in activating immune-mediated tumor killing. Because RT remains an effective means of inducing cell death and providing tumor antigen to the immune system, the use of RT in combination with immunotherapy has been studied in preclinical and clinical settings.[51,63–65]

Most of the recent studies that have validated RT as an effective partner for immunotherapy in preclinical and clinical settings have used immunotherapies that block T-cell checkpoint regulatory molecules. Such molecules include antibodies, such as anti–CTLA-4 and anti-PD1, which block inhibitory signals on T cells to unleash full T-cell effector function[63–65] and anti-OX40, an agonistic antibodies that target OX40 and costimulatory molecules that present for a short period after antigen stimulation. Costimulatory ligation results in proliferation of antigen-stimulated T cells,[66,67] including tumor-specific T cells, triggering their differentiation into effector and memory T cells with antitumor potential.[29] Recently the authors performed a pilot study of stereotactic body RT (SBRT) followed by high-dose IL-2, a potent proinflammatory cytokine, to assess safety and tumor response and to study immune monitoring in patients with metastatic melanoma or renal cell carcinoma.[68] Immune monitoring demonstrated a significantly higher frequency of proliferating $CD4^+$ T cells and an early activated effector memory phenotype in the peripheral blood of responding patients. Of patients in the trial, 67% responded to hypofractionated radiation followed by IL-2 compared with 15% of historical cohorts with IL-2 alone.

The rationale for this approach is that the addition of non-lymphotoxic doses of radiation will improve on the roughly 15% systemic response rate seen with anti–PD-1 alone. The proposed mechanism is a radiation-induced in situ vaccine effect, which propagates via epitope spreading to enhance antitumor immunity or, alternatively, via a local response that is dependent on blockade of upregulated PD-L1 in the tumor. PD-L1 upregulation following radiation has been shown to limit local tumor control in mouse models while blockade of PD-1/PD-L1 in combination with radiation have been shown to improve tumor control.

Investigators are interested in clinical trials studying the safety, efficacy, and sequencing of combining RT and various immunotherapy agents in many types of tumors, including HNSCC.[69] Well-designed, prospective trials will help determine the optimal dose, technique, and sequencing of RT with immunotherapies. Development of biomarkers to predict treatment response to immunotherapies will help identify patients most likely to benefit from various treatments. Despite the paucity of evidence showing the clinical safety and efficacy of combining RT with immunotherapy, the approach has the exciting potential of synergism to result in a more consistent abscopal effect. These encouraging preclinical and clinical results have led to a clinical trial under way at our institution to translate this approach for patients with HNSCC in the *definitive* setting (NCT03247712).

## CHEMOTHERAPY AND IMMUNOTHERAPY

Several molecular mechanisms have been identified by which chemotherapy may augment immune response against tumor cells. First, inducing immunogenic tumor cell death results in the release of tumor antigens, which are presented by DCs, and molecular signals, such as damage-associated molecular patterns (DAMPs) that cumulatively engage the immune system.[70] Second, the expression of formyl peptide receptor 1 on DCs favors stable interactions with annexin-1–expressing dying cancer cells, DC maturation, and cross-presentation of TAAs.[71] Third, homeostasis and inhibition are disrupted in the function of T-reg lymphocytes.

Although several clinical trials have investigated combinations of chemotherapy and checkpoint blockade, most studies were primarily designed to detect differences between groups receiving chemotherapy alone versus chemotherapy plus checkpoint blockade. Combination therapy and immunotherapy alone have not been directly compared, making difficult the accurate assessment of the effect of the chemotherapy component to the combination arms. Early reports from the Checkmate 012 study investigating 4 different combinations of platinum-based chemotherapy with the anti–PD-1 antibody nivolumab indicated that none of the arms had a median progression-free survival exceeding that observed for nivolumab alone.[72]

## SURGERY AND IMMUNOTHERAPY

Cytoreductive surgery aims to reduce the number of cancer cells via resection of primary tumor or metastatic deposits, in an effort to minimize a potentially immunosuppressive tumor burden, palliate symptoms, and prevent complications. Furthermore, specimens provide a platform for investigation of biomarkers to optimize immunotherapy, to reverse the immunosuppressive TME, and to enhance adaptive immune response.[73]

In mice models, Gough and colleagues[51] have shown that surgical removal of a large primary sarcoma results in local recurrence in approximately 50% of animals. Depletion of CD8 T cells resulted in local recurrence in 100% of animals, indicating that these cells were involved in the control of residual disease. The systemic adjuvant administration of anti-OX40 at surgery eliminated local recurrences. In this model, anti-OX40 acted to directly enhance tumor antigen-specific CD8 T-cell proliferation in the lymph node draining the surgical site, and resulted in increased tumor antigen-specific cytotoxicity in vivo. A phase Ib clinical trial using anti-OX40 (MEDI6469) at various dose intervals before definitive surgical resection of patients with HNSCC is currently under way (NCT02274155).[60]

Recently, the authors demonstrated that activating intratumoral cyclic dinucleotide (CDN) ligand of the stimulator of interferon genes (STING) pathway strongly induces type I IFN and TNFα, resulting in rapid regression in a range of HNSCC tumor models.[74] We developed a novel intervention using a biomaterial containing CDN ligands (STINGblade), which is implanted locally into the resection site at the time of surgery and prevents local recurrence following subtotal surgical resection. In a series of experiments using 2 different models of HNSCC, we showed that this antitumor activity was STING- and CD8-dependent, suggesting that adaptive immune responses are required for control of disease and improved survival. We hold great hope for this combination strategy personalized to target immune-suppressive mechanisms in the TME.

## SUMMARY AND FUTURE DIRECTIONS

Recently, immunotherapy with checkpoint inhibitors targeting PD-1 were approved by the FDA for use in HNSCC based on data that showed improved OS in patients with recurrent metastatic disease.[4,5] However, response rates were as low as 13% to 20% and durable tumor remission occurred in few patients. One possible explanation for this observation is that some HNSCCs cause alterations in the generation, processing, and/or presentation of T-cell epitopes derived from TAAs by human leukocyte antigen (HLA) class I and/or class II molecules and cannot generate an effective immune response.[75] Alternatively, some patients with cancer generate effector immune cells, yet tumors persist through adaptation and natural selection of clonal cancer cell populations, which then evade immune recognition and clearance through various mechanisms, such as T-cell exhaustion (eg, loss of HLA expression or defects in antigen-processing machinery), upregulation of inhibitory immune checkpoint pathways (eg, PD-1/PD-L1),[76] alterations in signal transduction pathways (eg, JAK1/2),[77] the presence of immune-suppressive cells (eg, T-regs, myeloid-derived suppressor cells[78]), or secretion of immune-suppressive mediators (eg, TGF-beta).[79]

Over the past 5 years, the authors' research has used automated staining equipment, imaging devices, both scanners and imaging microscopes, as well as various software to assess digital images to chart significant advances. We have applied mIHC to evaluate a cohort of 119 patients with HPV-HNSCC. Although stratification based on CD8 T-cell numbers showed a significant prognostic biomarker, enumeration of tumors for FoxP3+ or PD-L1+ cells (high or low) did not provide a prognostic significance. Nonetheless, when considering geography of the microenvironment, we found a striking correlation between the number of FoxP3+ T cells within 30 μm of CD8 T cells and the number of PD-L1+ cells within 30 μm of CD8 T cells, and patient survival. The implications question the relevance of other tissue-based biomarker assays that do not consider distance (eg, single-stain immunohistochemistry for PDL-1), and support the significance of CSI. The findings also underscore the importance of performing immunologic biomarker studies on biopsies at initial cancer diagnosis in correlation with changes in the tumor and draining lymph nodes.

The induction of T-cell immunity is crucial to successful cancer immunotherapy. Tumor biomarker studies of immune cells infiltrating the tumor or tumor margin, as well as immune-related gene profiles of patients being treated with checkpoint blockade, suggest that patients who have a preexisting or endogenous immune response have a better outcome than patients lacking this activated "inflamed phenotype." Nonetheless, many patients generate immune responses to antigen, but do not respond to conventional treatment or immunotherapy.

Multiple strategies for initiating an effective immune response are under investigation. In addition to the STING pathway reviewed previously, therapeutic vaccines have been used to induce broad humoral immunity to the spectrum of TAA that are overexpressed in a given tumor (eg, whole-cell vaccines). However, because the TAAs are "shared" with normal cells and may trigger central and peripheral tolerance mechanisms leading to the selection of T cells with low-affinity TCRs, the effectiveness of these vaccines has been limited to date. Alternatively, tumor-specific neoantigens, which arise via mutations that alter amino acid coding sequences (nonsynonymous somatic mutations) have emerged as promising targets for T-cell–directed immunotherapy. Because normal tissues do not express these somatic mutations, neoantigen-specific T cells are not subject to central and peripheral tolerance. The therapeutic efficacy of either approach remains to be determined. Likewise, the effect of surgical removal of TAA or neoantigens on subsequent immune response is yet unknown. Answers to these key questions and the development of biomarkers that predict the response to conventional treatment modalities and immunotherapy offer great promise to the field of oncology and focus for ongoing investigation in T-cell–directed immunotherapy.

Currently, patients who fail conventional therapies and immunotherapy have few treatment options. As treatment with immunotherapy continues to increase, an emerging challenge in patients with recurrent metastatic HNSCC will be progression of disease while under treatment with checkpoint inhibitors. Defining ongoing tumor-specific T-cell response at the molecular level for individual patients strives to identify strategies of boosting tumor antigen-specific T-cell responses in these patients. The individualized data of such investigation could amplify the endogenous T-cell response and thereby develop specific personalized treatments for patients with recurrent disease.

One approach under investigation for personalized immunotherapy is adoptive transfer of T cells engineered to respond to specific mutated epitopes, or neoantigens. By this method, TCRs are isolated from TIL in an individual patient and next-generation sequencing is performed on tumor cells of the same patient to identify the expression of nonsynonymous mutations (**Fig. 5**).[80–82] Each mutation is then encoded into minigene constructs, which are then linked in tandem to generate a tandem minigene (TMG) construct that can be used in a semi–high-throughput method of evaluating the immunogenicity of mutations. These TMG constructs are then introduced into autologous DCs, processed, and presented in the context of the patient's own HLA class I and II molecules. Retroviral supernatants encoding each one of the TCRs are generated and used to transduce autologous T cells. Any reactive TCRs identified are tested against the wild-type peptide to determine whether the TCR is neoantigen-specific. Neoantigen-specific T cells are then expanded ex vivo and infused into the patient in combination with high-dose IL-1. This approach has been

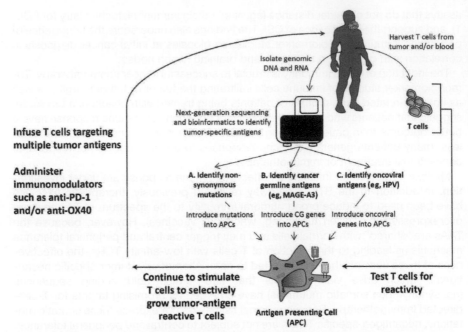

**Fig. 5.** Adoptive T-cell therapy targeting neoantigens. Traditional adoptive T-cell therapy involves harvesting T cells from autologous tumor resection or biopsy, expanding them ex vivo with IL-2, testing for tumor specificity, and then rapidly expanding them for reinfusion into a nonmyeloablative lymphodepleted patient, usually with concurrently high-dose IL-2. One approach under investigation for personalized immunotherapy is to adoptively transfer T cells engineered to respond to specific mutated epitopes, or neoantigens.

used successfully in upper aerodigestive tract malignancy and offers a promising strategy for patients with HNSCC.

In conclusion, a minority of patients with HNSCC will respond and benefit from anti–PD-1 and other immunotherapies as monotherapy. To advance the field of immunotherapy, future trials must vigorously integrate conventional therapies, such as surgery, radiation, and chemotherapy, combine immunotherapies in rational sequences for patients with immune responsiveness, and develop novel, personalized therapeutic approaches for patients lacking an effective immune response. A new era of immunotherapy awaits with high optimism for improving outcomes in patients with HNSCC.

## REFERENCES

1. Cooper JS, Pajak TF, Forastiere AA, et al. Postoperative concurrent radiotherapy and chemotherapy for high-risk squamous-cell carcinoma of the head and neck. N Engl J Med 2004;350(19):1937–44.

2. Bernier J, Domenge C, Ozsahin M, et al. Postoperative irradiation with or without concomitant chemotherapy for locally advanced head and neck cancer. N Engl J Med 2004;350(19):1945–52.

3. Ang KK, Harris J, Wheeler R, et al. Human papillomavirus and survival of patients with oropharyngeal cancer. N Engl J Med 2010;363(1):24–35.

4. Seiwert TY, Burtness B, Mehra R, et al. Safety and clinical activity of pembrolizumab for treatment of recurrent or metastatic squamous cell carcinoma of the

head and neck (KEYNOTE-012): an open-label, multicentre, phase 1b trial. Lancet Oncol 2016;17(7):956–65.

5. Ferris RL, Blumenschein G, Fayette J, et al. Nivolumab for recurrent squamous-cell carcinoma of the head and neck. N Engl J Med 2016;375(19):1856–67.

6. Prehn RT, Main JM. Immunity to methylcholanthrene-induced sarcomas. J Natl Cancer Inst 1957;18(6):769–78.

7. Burnet FM. Immunological aspects of malignant disease. Lancet 1967;1(7501): 1171–4.

8. Duhen T, Duhen R, Montler R, et al. Co-expression of CD39 and CD103 identifies tumor-reactive CD8 T cells in human solid tumors. Nat Commun 2018;9(1):2724.

9. Mittal D, Gubin MM, Schreiber RD, et al. New insights into cancer immunoediting and its three component phases—elimination, equilibrium and escape. Curr Opin Immunol 2014;27:16–25.

10. Gajewski TF. The next hurdle in cancer immunotherapy: overcoming the non-T-cell-inflamed tumor microenvironment. Semin Oncol 2015;42(4):663–71.

11. Feng Z, Bethmann D, Kappler M, et al. Multi-parametric immune profiling in HPV-negative oral squamous cell cancer. JCI Insight 2017;2(14) [pii:93652]. PMC5518563.

12. Albers AE, Strauss L, Liao T, et al. T cell-tumor interaction directs the development of immunotherapies in head and neck cancer. Clin Dev Immunol 2010; 2010:236378.

13. Ward MJ, Thirdborough SM, Mellows T, et al. Tumour-infiltrating lymphocytes predict for outcome in HPV-positive oropharyngeal cancer. Br J Cancer 2014;110(2): 489–500.

14. Green VL, Michno A, Stafford ND, et al. Increased prevalence of tumour infiltrating immune cells in oropharyngeal tumours in comparison to other subsites: relationship to peripheral immunity. Cancer Immunol Immunother 2013;62(5): 863–73.

15. Wansom D, Light E, Worden F, et al. Correlation of cellular immunity with human papillomavirus 16 status and outcome in patients with advanced oropharyngeal cancer. Arch Otolaryngol Head Neck Surg 2010;136(12):1267–73.

16. Grizzle WE, Xu X, Zhang S, et al. Age-related increase of tumor susceptibility is associated with myeloid-derived suppressor cell mediated suppression of T cell cytotoxicity in recombinant inbred BXD12 mice. Mech Ageing Dev 2007; 128(11–12):672–80.

17. Yang W, Chen PW, Li H, et al. PD-L1: PD-1 interaction contributes to the functional suppression of T-cell responses to human uveal melanoma cells in vitro. Invest Ophthalmol Vis Sci 2008;49(6):2518–25.

18. Brahmer JR, Drake CG, Wollner I, et al. Phase I study of single-agent anti-programmed death-1 (MDX-1106) in refractory solid tumors: safety, clinical activity, pharmacodynamics, and immunologic correlates. J Clin Oncol 2010;28(19): 3167–75.

19. Varilla V, Atienza J, Dasanu CA. Immune alterations and immunotherapy prospects in head and neck cancer. Expert Opin Biol Ther 2013;13(9):1241–56.

20. Baruah P, Lee M, Odutoye T, et al. Decreased levels of alternative co-stimulatory receptors OX40 and 4-1BB characterise T cells from head and neck cancer patients. Immunobiology 2012;217(7):669–75.

21. Badoual C, Hans S, Merillon N, et al. PD-1-expressing tumor-infiltrating T cells are a favorable prognostic biomarker in HPV-associated head and neck cancer. Cancer Res 2013;73(1):128–38.

22. Rubin Grandis J, Melhem MF, Gooding WE, et al. Levels of TGF-alpha and EGFR protein in head and neck squamous cell carcinoma and patient survival. J Natl Cancer Inst 1998;90(11):824–32.
23. Bonner JA, Harari PM, Giralt J, et al. Radiotherapy plus cetuximab for squamous-cell carcinoma of the head and neck. N Engl J Med 2006;354(6):567–78.
24. Vermorken JB, Mesia R, Rivera F, et al. Platinum-based chemotherapy plus cetuximab in head and neck cancer. N Engl J Med 2008;359(11):1116–27.
25. Gildener-Leapman N, Ferris RL, Bauman JE. Promising systemic immunotherapies in head and neck squamous cell carcinoma. Oral Oncol 2013;49(12): 1089–96.
26. Curtsinger JM, Schmidt CS, Mondino A, et al. Inflammatory cytokines provide a third signal for activation of naive CD4+ and CD8+ T cells. J Immunol 1999; 162(6):3256–62.
27. Guntermann C, Alexander DR. CTLA-4 suppresses proximal TCR signaling in resting human CD4(+) T cells by inhibiting ZAP-70 Tyr(319) phosphorylation: a potential role for tyrosine phosphatases. J Immunol 2002;168(9):4420–9.
28. Romano E, Kusio-Kobialka M, Foukas PG, et al. Ipilimumab-dependent cell-mediated cytotoxicity of regulatory T cells ex vivo by nonclassical .monocytes in melanoma patients. Proc Natl Acad Sci U S A 2015;112(19):6140–5.
29. Weinberg AD, Rivera MM, Prell R, et al. Engagement of the OX-40 receptor in vivo enhances antitumor immunity. J Immunol 2000;164(4):2160–9.
30. Hodi FS, O'Day SJ, McDermott DF, et al. Improved survival with ipilimumab in patients with metastatic melanoma. N Engl J Med 2010;363(8):711–23.
31. Sheppard K-A, Fitz LJ, Lee JM, et al. PD-1 inhibits T-cell receptor induced phosphorylation of the ZAP70/CD3zeta signalosome and downstream signaling to PKCtheta. FEBS Lett 2004;574(1–3):37–41.
32. Iwai Y, Terawaki S, Honjo T. PD-1 blockade inhibits hematogenous spread of poorly immunogenic tumor cells by enhanced recruitment of effector T cells. Int Immunol 2005;17(2):133–44.
33. Nomi T, Sho M, Akahori T, et al. Clinical significance and therapeutic potential of the programmed death-1 ligand/programmed death-1 pathway in human pancreatic cancer. Clin Cancer Res 2007;13(7):2151–7.
34. Mangsbo SM, Sandin LC, Anger K, et al. Enhanced tumor eradication by combining CTLA-4 or PD-1 blockade with CpG therapy. J Immunother 2010; 33(3):225–35.
35. Callahan MK, Kluger H, Postow MA, et al. Nivolumab plus Ipilimumab in patients with advanced melanoma: updated survival, response, and safety data in a phase I dose-escalation study. J Clin Oncol 2018;36(4):391–8.
36. Lipson EJ, Sharfman WH, Drake CG, et al. Durable cancer regression off-treatment and effective reinduction therapy with an anti-PD-1 antibody. Clin Cancer Res 2013;19(2):462–8.
37. Topalian SL, Hodi FS, Brahmer JR, et al. Safety, activity, and immune correlates of anti-PD-1 antibody in cancer. N Engl J Med 2012;366(26):2443–54.
38. Wolchok JD, Chiarion-Sileni V, Gonzalez R, et al. Overall survival with combined nivolumab and ipilimumab in advanced melanoma. N Engl J Med 2017;377(14): 1345–56.
39. Larkins E, Blumenthal GM, Yuan W, et al. FDA approval summary: pembrolizumab for the treatment of recurrent or metastatic head and neck squamous cell carcinoma with disease progression on or after platinum-containing chemotherapy. Oncologist 2017;22(7):873–8.

40. Cohen EE, Harrington KJ, Le Tourneau C, et al. Pembrolizumab (pembro) vs standard of care (SOC) for recurrent or metastatic head and neck squamous cell carcinoma (R/M HNSCC): phase 3 KEYNOTE-040 trial. Ann Oncol 2017;28(suppl_5): 628.

41. Freeman GJ, Long AJ, Iwai Y, et al. Engagement of the PD-1 immunoinhibitory receptor by a novel B7 family member leads to negative regulation of lymphocyte activation. J Exp Med 2000;192(7):1027–34.

42. Chen J, Feng Y, Lu L, et al. Interferon-γ-induced PD-L1 surface expression on human oral squamous carcinoma via PKD2 signal pathway. Immunobiology 2012; 217(4):385–93.

43. Akbay EA, Koyama S, Carretero J, et al. Activation of the PD-1 pathway contributes to immune escape in EGFR-driven lung tumors. Cancer Discov 2013;3(12): 1355–63.

44. Terawaki S, Chikuma S, Shibayama S, et al. IFN-α directly promotes programmed cell death-1 transcription and limits the duration of T cell-mediated immunity. J Immunol 2011;186(5):2772–9.

45. Brahmer JR, Tykodi SS, Chow LQM, et al. Safety and activity of anti-PD-L1 antibody in patients with advanced cancer. N Engl J Med 2012;366(26):2455–65.

46. Innate pharma provides an update on Lirilumab. Available at: http://www.innate-pharma. com/en/news-events/press-releases/innate-pharma-provides-update-lirilumab. Accessed February 18, 2018.

47. Melero I, Shuford WW, Newby SA, et al. Monoclonal antibodies against the 4-1BB T-cell activation molecule eradicate established tumors. Nat Med 1997;3(6): 682–5.

48. Montler R, Bell RB, Thalhofer C, et al. OX40, PD-1 and CTLA-4 are selectively expressed on tumor-infiltrating T cells in head and neck cancer. Clin Transl Immunology 2016;5(4):e70.

49. Bell RB, Leidner RS, Crittenden MR, et al. OX40 signaling in head and neck squamous cell carcinoma: overcoming immunosuppression in the tumor microenvironment. Oral Oncol 2016;52:1–10.

50. Jensen SM, Maston LD, Gough MJ, et al. Signaling through OX40 enhances antitumor immunity. Semin Oncol 2010;37(5):524–32.

51. Gough MJ, Crittenden MR, Sarff M, et al. Adjuvant therapy with agonistic antibodies to CD134 (OX40) increases local control after surgical or radiation therapy of cancer in mice. J Immunother 2010;33(8):798–809.

52. Curti BD, Kovacsovics-Bankowski M, Morris N, et al. OX40 is a potent immune-stimulating target in late-stage cancer patients. Cancer Res 2013;73(24): 7189–98.

53. Cheuk ATC, Mufti GJ, Guinn B-A. Role of 4-1BB:4-1BB ligand in cancer immunotherapy. Cancer Gene Ther 2004;11(3):215–26.

54. Mittler RS, Bailey TS, Klussman K, et al. Anti-4-1BB monoclonal antibodies abrogate T cell-dependent humoral immune responses in vivo through the induction of helper T cell anergy. J Exp Med 1999;190(10):1535–40.

55. Bartkowiak T, Curran MA. 4-1BB agonists: multi-potent potentiators of tumor immunity. Front Oncol 2015;5:117.

56. Rosenberg SA, Yang JC, Sherry RM, et al. Durable complete responses in heavily pretreated patients with metastatic melanoma using T-cell transfer immunotherapy. Clin Cancer Res 2011;17(13):4550–7.

57. Ohtani T, Yamada Y, Furuhashi A, et al. Activated cytotoxic T-lymphocyte immunotherapy is effective for advanced oral and maxillofacial cancers. Int J Oncol 2014;45(5):2051–7.

58. Chacon JA, Sarnaik AA, Chen JQ, et al. Manipulating the tumor microenvironment ex vivo for enhanced expansion of tumor-infiltrating lymphocytes for adoptive cell therapy. Clin Cancer Res 2015;21(3):611–21.

59. Junker N, Andersen MH, Wenandy L, et al. Bimodal ex vivo expansion of T cells from patients with head and neck squamous cell carcinoma: a prerequisite for adoptive cell transfer. Cytotherapy 2011;13(7):822–34.

60. Bell RB, Duhen R, Leidner R, et al. Neoadjuvant anti-OX40 (MEDI6469) prior to surgery in head and neck squamous cell carcinoma. J Clin Oncol 2018; 36(suppl) [abstract: 6011].

61. Twitty CG, Jensen SM, Hu H-M, et al. Tumor-derived autophagosome vaccine: induction of cross-protective immune responses against short-lived proteins through a p62-dependent mechanism. Clin Cancer Res 2011;17(20):6467–81.

62. Usami Y, Ishida K, Sato S, et al. Intercellular adhesion molecule-1 (ICAM-1) expression correlates with oral cancer progression and induces macrophage/cancer cell adhesion. Int J Cancer 2013;133(3):568–78.

63. Twyman-Saint Victor C, Rech AJ, Maity A, et al. Radiation and dual checkpoint blockade activate non-redundant immune mechanisms in cancer. Nature 2015; 520(7547):373–7.

64. Pilones KA, Kawashima N, Yang AM, et al. Invariant natural killer T cells regulate breast cancer response to radiation and CTLA-4 blockade. Clin Cancer Res 2009;15(2):597–606.

65. Deng L, Liang H, Xu M, et al. STING-dependent cytosolic DNA sensing promotes radiation-induced type I interferon-dependent antitumor immunity in immunogenic tumors. Immunity 2014;41(5):843–52.

66. Redmond WL, Ruby CE, Weinberg AD. The role of OX40-mediated co-stimulation in T-cell activation and survival. Crit Rev Immunol 2009;29(3):187–201.

67. Ruby CE, Redmond WL, Haley D, et al. Anti-OX40 stimulation in vivo enhances CD8+ memory T cell survival and significantly increases recall responses. Eur J Immunol 2007;37(1):157–66.

68. Gough MJ, Killeen N, Weinberg AD. Targeting macrophages in the tumour environment to enhance the efficacy of αOX40 therapy. Immunology 2012;136(4): 437–47.

69. Kang J, Demaria S, Formenti S. Current clinical trials testing the combination of immunotherapy with radiotherapy. J Immunother Cancer 2016;4:51.

70. Krysko DV, Garg AD, Kaczmarek A, et al. Immunogenic cell death and DAMPs in cancer therapy. Nat Rev Cancer 2012;12(12):860–75.

71. Vacchelli E, Ma Y, Baracco EE, et al. Chemotherapy-induced antitumor immunity requires formyl peptide receptor 1. Science 2015;350(6263):972–8.

72. Antonia SJ, Brahmer JR, Gettinger S, et al. Nivolumab (Anti-PD-1; BMS-936558, ONO-4538) in combination with platinum-based doublet chemotherapy (PT-DC) in advanced non-small cell lung cancer (NSCLC): metastatic non-small cell lung cancer. Int J Radiat Oncol Biol Phys 2014;90(5):S2.

73. Bell RB, Gough MJ, Seung SK, et al. Cytoreductive surgery for head and neck squamous cell carcinoma in the new age of immunotherapy. Oral Oncol 2016; 61:166–76.

74. Baird JR, Feng Z, Xiao HD, et al. STING expression and response to treatment with STING ligands in premalignant and malignant disease. PLoS One 2017; 12(11):e0187532.

75. Tran E, Ahmadzadeh M, Lu YC, et al. Immunogenicity of somatic mutations in human gastrointestinal cancers. Science 2015;350:1387–90.

76. Sanghoon Shin D, Zaretsky JM, Escuin-Ordinas H, et al. Primary resistance to PD-1 blockade mediated by JAK1/2 mutations. Cancer Discov 2017;7(2): 188–201.

77. Spranger S, Spaapen RM, Zha Y, et al. Up-regulation of PD-L1, IDO, and Tregs in the melanoma tumor microenvironment is driven by CD+ T cells. Sci Transl Med 2013;5(200):200ra116.

78. Jie HB, Gildener-Leapman N, Li J, et al. Intratumoral regulatory T cells upregulate immunosuppressive molecules in head and neck cancer patients. Br J Cancer 2013;109:2629–35.

79. Gordon SR, Maute RL, Dulken BW, et al. PD-1 expression by tumour-associated macrophages inhibits phagocytosis and tumour immunity. Nature 2017; 545(7655):495–9.

80. Tran E, Robbins PF, Lu YC, et al. T-cell transfer therapy targeting mutant KRAS in cancer. N Engl J Med 2016;375(23):2255–62.

81. Tran E, Robbins PF, Rosenberg SA. 'Final common pathway' of human cancer immunotherapy: targeting random somatic mutations. Nat Immunol 2017;18: 255–62.

82. Tran E, Turcotte S, Gros A, et al. Cancer immunotherapy based on mutation-specific CD4+ T cells in a patient with epithelial cancer. Science 2014;344:641–5.

# The Current Status of Immunotherapies in Esophagogastric Cancer

Geoffrey Y. Ku, MD

## KEYWORDS

- Adenocarcinoma • Squamous cell carcinoma • Gastric • Esophageal
- Immunotherapy • Immune checkpoint • PD-1 • PD-L1

## KEY POINTS

- Immune checkpoint inhibitors that target cytotoxic T lymphocyte antigen-4 or the programmed death-1/programmed death–ligand 1 axis have transformed the treatment of many solid tumors.
- Initial phase I/II studies in esophagogastric cancer suggest significant activity for these drugs.
- Ongoing phase III studies will determine if there is a role for these drugs in the next several years.
- Correlative analyses are ongoing to identify the group of patients most likely to benefit from these therapies.

## INTRODUCTION

Outcomes for patients with advanced esophagogastric cancer (EGC) are poor.[1] Approximately 50% of patients with EGC present with overt metastatic disease, and chemotherapy is the mainstay of palliation in this setting. With the high likelihood that patients with initial locoregional disease will eventually have metastatic disease, palliative chemotherapy will ultimately be used in most patients. In recent years, the incorporation of targeted agents—trastuzumab with first-line chemotherapy for Her2-positive disease[2] and ramucirumab as monotherapy[3] or with paclitaxel chemotherapy[4] in the second-line setting—has incrementally improved outcomes, but median overall survival (OS) remains at best only 1 year.

In this gloomy context, excitement is growing among oncologists and patients alike for the use of immunotherapy or, more specifically, immune checkpoint inhibitors.

This article originally appeared in *Surgical Oncology Clinics of North America*, Volume 26, Issue 2, April 2017.

Disclosure: Dr G.Y. Ku received research support from Merck and AstraZeneca/Medimmune.

Gastrointestinal Oncology Service, Department of Medicine, Memorial Sloan Kettering Cancer Center, 300 East 66th Street, Room 1035, New York, NY 10065, USA

*E-mail address:* kug@mskcc.org

Hematol Oncol Clin N Am 33 (2019) 323–338
https://doi.org/10.1016/j.hoc.2018.12.007
0889-8588/19/© 2018 Elsevier Inc. All rights reserved.

Since the landmark approval by the US Food and Drug Administration (FDA) of the anti–cytotoxic T-lymphocyte antigen-4 (CTLA-4) antibody ipilimumab in advanced melanoma,[5,6] these and other antibodies (namely, antagonists of the programmed death [PD]-1/PD-ligand 1 pathway) that de-repress the immune system have undergone extensive evaluation in multiple other solid tumors, including EGC. These studies have led to the FDA approval of additional immune checkpoint inhibitors in several solid tumor malignancies and, in EGC, have culminated in ongoing phase III studies.

This review focuses on the role of the immune system in cancer, a brief history of immunotherapy, the role of immune checkpoint molecules in normal immune homeostasis and, the rapidly accumulating data in EGC.

## THE IMMUNE SYSTEM

The immune system protects us from external threats (infectious diseases) and also from internal ones (cancers) while not attacking healthy tissue (which would lead to the development of autoimmune diseases). To fulfill these critical and synchronous roles, it must recognize self from non–self-antigens with unerring accuracy.

The immune system consists of an innate and an adaptive component.[7] The innate immune system involves rapid immune responses, which are mediated by macrophages, neutrophils, dendritic cells, and natural killer cells. These cells are hard wired to recognize non–self-antigens, such as those from infectious organisms, but have (1) relatively low potency, (2) limited specificity for the specific microorganism, and (3) no memory (ie, no ability to generate an enhanced response if re-exposed to the same microorganism).

If a microbe or cancer cell is not rapidly eliminated by innate immune mechanisms, adaptive immune responses are then engendered. These responses are produced by B cells (the humoral arm, which produces antibodies that typically target extracellular antigens) and T cells (the cellular arm, which destroys infected cells that harbor intracellular organisms or malignant cells). In contrast to innate immunity, adaptive immunity develops over days to weeks and is (1) much more potent, (2) highly specific for a specific antigen, and (3) leads to a memory response (which results in a much more rapid and potent response upon re-exposure).

Despite these coordinated mechanisms, the development of cancer necessarily implies a failure of immunosurveillance of incipient malignant cells. Dunn and colleagues[8] proposed the concept of immunoediting to explain this phenomenon. They envisaged that this process comprises 3 phases that are collectively denoted as the 3 Es of cancer immunoediting: elimination, equilibrium, and escape. The first E refers to the fact that most cancer cells are indeed recognized and successfully killed by the immune system, leading to the second E, where the surviving cancer cells acquire multiple mechanisms that allow them to exist alongside increasingly ineffective immune responses (eg, downregulating immunogenic molecules on the tumor cell surface or recruiting immunosuppressive mechanisms in the tumor microenvironment). This second E lasts the longest and may occur over many years. Finally, the balance of forces shifts decidedly in the favor of the cancer cells, allowing them to escape from immune control.

## COLEY'S TOXINS

The idea of harnessing the immune system to attack cancer is an intuitively appealing concept but not a new one. The attractiveness of such a proposed treatment stems from the belief that recruitment of the immune system to attack cancer cells potentially offers more durable benefit and less toxicity than conventional therapies (akin to fighting off a virulent influenza infection) and, in some fashion, is more natural than the harsh chemicals and x-rays that comprise modern anticancer therapy.

The earliest proof of the potential of the immune system to directly combat malignant tumors stems from a series of observations and experiments by William Coley, a surgeon at the New York Cancer Hospital (the precursor to Memorial Sloan Kettering Cancer Center).[9] He noted the regression of a soft tissue sarcoma in a patient who had erysipelas, an infection caused by *Streptococcus pyogenes*. He then inoculated the tumors of 10 patients directly with a culture of the bacterium and noted durable curative responses in some patients. The immune basis of these observations is not known with certainty but is presumed to involve the nonspecific recruitment to the tumor site and activation of immune cells by the bacterial products.[10]

Although Coley's concoction of toxins fell out of favor, other approaches to stimulate the immune system continued to be investigated in the 20th century. Most of these methods focused on vaccinating patients against preidentified antigens that are expressed preferentially or exclusively on tumor cells.[11] Uniformly, despite laboratory evidence of cellular immune responses to these vaccines, few clinically relevant responses were noted.

The sole exception is sipuleucel-T, a recombinant human protein consisting of prostatic acid phosphatase linked to granulocyte-macrophage colony-stimulating factor, which has to be introduced into autologous peripheral blood mononuclear cells obtained from patients by leukopheresis. It was approved in 2010 for the treatment of castrate-resistant prostate cancer based on a phase III study, which found an improvement in OS in the absence of an improvement in time to progression.[12]

The low effectiveness of most cancer vaccines is likely because of their lack of antigenicity and the failure to provide adequate costimulation (to be discussed later), which results in inactivation of T cells against the tumor.[13]

## IMMUNE CHECKPOINTS

The generation of an effective cellular immune response by T cells against a cancer cell requires a primary signal and cosignals.[14] As shown in **Fig. 1**, the primary signal comes from recognition of a cancer-associated antigen by a T-cell receptor with high specificity for the antigen, presented in the context of a class I/II major histocompatibility complex molecule, which is expressed on so-called antigen-present cells (APCs), such as dendritic cells or on the tumor cell itself. In addition to this primary signal, a secondary signal is required, in the absence of which the T cell may be rendered anergic or nonfunctional.

As noted in **Fig. 1**, it is now well established that the interactions between multiple molecules at the interface between the T cell and tumor cell create multiple secondary signals, some of which are costimulatory and some of which are inhibitory. The ultimate activation or quiescence of the immune response depends on the complex interplay and net signal—positive or negative—of these diverse interactions, which occur at different times in the process of successful T-cell engagement and activation.

Under normal physiologic conditions, immune checkpoints are crucial for the maintenance of self-tolerance (and the avoidance of autoimmunity) and also to protect tissues from excessive damage if the immune system were to respond too exuberantly to an infection. However, many of these molecules have become co-opted by cancer cells (in the process of achieving equilibrium and escape from the immune system). Their identification and targeting with neutralizing (or agonist) antibodies now forms the basis of modern-era immunotherapy.

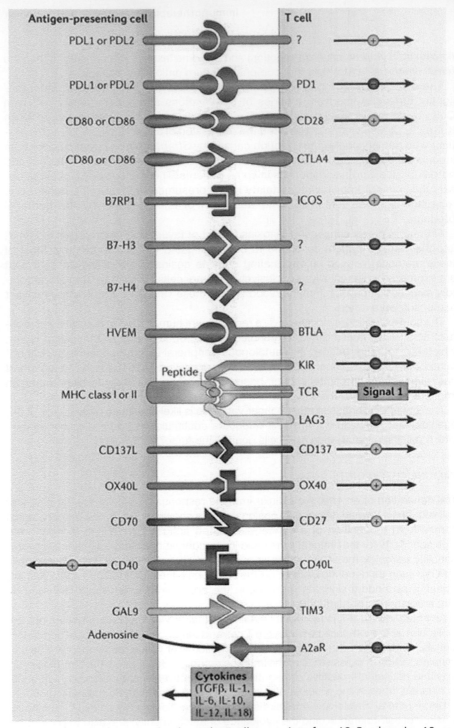

**Fig. 1.** Immune checkpoint molecules at the T cell–tumor interface. A2aR, adenosine A2a receptor; B7RP1, B7-related protein 1; BTLA, B and T lymphocyte attenuator; GAL9, galectin 9; HVEM, herpesvirus entry mediator; ICOS, inducible T-cell costimulator; IL, interleukin; KIR, killer cell immunoglobulinlike receptor; LAG3, lymphocyte activation gene 3; PD1, programmed cell death protein 1; PDL, PD1 ligand; TGFβ, transforming growth factor-β; TIM3, T cell membrane protein 3. (*From* Pardoll DM. The blockade of immune checkpoints in cancer immunotherapy. Nat Rev Cancer 2012;12:252; with permission.)

## Cytotoxic T-Lymphocyte Antigen-4 and the Programmed Death-1/Programmed Death–ligand 1/2 Pathway

In 1995, James Allison and colleagues[15] were 1 of 2 groups that simultaneously characterized the function of CTLA-4, a protein that has high homology with CD28, which was already known to be a costimulatory molecule expressed on T cells necessary to provide the secondary signal for T-cell activation. Just like CD28, CTLA-4 also binds their cognate ligands, the B7 molecules (which are found on APCs), but with much higher affinity. However, unlike CD28, CTLA-4 expression is induced only when a T cell becomes activated. It then competes with CD28 for binding to the B7 molecules but leads to down-regulation and eventual abrogation of the immune response.

Subsequently, PD-1 was also identified as another negative immune checkpoint molecule.[16] PD-1 has 2 ligands, PD-L1 and PD-L2. PD-L2 is mostly expressed on APCs, whereas PD-L1 is expressed on numerous tissues, including immune and tumor cells. In the tumor microenvironment, PD-L1 expressed on tumor cells binds to PD-1 on activated T cells reaching the tumor. This delivers an inhibitory signal to those T cells, preventing them from killing target cancer cells and protecting the tumor from immune elimination.[17] Unlike CTLA-4, which is thought to be necessary for T-cell activation, the PD-1/PD-L1/2 pathway is thought to protect cells from T-cell attack.[18]

## Anti–Cytotoxic T-Lymphocyte Antigen-4 Antibodies

The 2 anti–CTLA-4 antibodies that have been evaluated in EGC are ipilimumab and tremelimumab. In the first-line phase III study of ipilimumab in advanced melanoma, immune-related adverse events (irAEs) resulted from nonspecific immune activation and included diarrhea (33% all grade, 4% grade 3), pruritus (27% all grade, 2% grade 3), rash (22% all grade, 1.2% grade 3), and elevation in liver enzymes (about 29% all grade, 15% grade 3/4).[6] No treatment-related deaths were reported. Since that time, the growing clinical experience with ipilimumab and other immune checkpoint inhibitors has also led to well-established algorithms for treating irAEs with the use of steroids and other immunosuppressants, which do not appear to reduce the benefit from ipilimumab in melanoma patients.[19]

Historically, the first immune checkpoint inhibitor to be studied in EGC was tremelimumab. In a phase II study, Ralph and colleagues[20] evaluated tremelimumab, 15 mg/kg every 90 days, in 18 patients with advanced esophageal, gastroesophageal junction (GEJ), or gastric adenocarcinoma; 15 received prior first-line chemotherapy, and 3 received prior second-line treatment. One patient achieved a partial response (PR, 6%) by standard Response Evaluation Criteria in Solid Tumors (RECIST) criteria that was ongoing at 33 months of follow-up, whereas 4 other patients achieved stable disease (SD, 22%). Although median time to progression and OS were disappointing (2.83 and 4.83 months respectively), one-third of patients were alive at 12 months. Grade $\geq 3$ toxicities included rash and diarrhea in 2 and 3 patients, respectively, consistent with the known toxicities of these drugs. Correlative analyses included evaluating T-cell proliferative responses to carcinoembryonic antigen; the 5 patients with a posttreatment response had improved OS compared with the 8 assayed patients without a carcinoembryonic antigen response (17.1 vs 4.7 months; $P = .004$).

The dose of tremelimumab in this study is now considered subtherapeutic. In an ongoing study of tremelimumab (with or without the anti–PD-L1 antibody, durvalumab), the dose of tremelimumab monotherapy is 10 mg/kg every 4 weeks.

Data for ipilimumab were recently reported in abstract form.[21] This was for a randomized phase II study in which 114 patients with either a PR or SD to first-line fluoropyrimidine/platinum chemotherapy were randomly assigned to best supportive care

(BSC, which mostly consisted of continuation of the fluoropyrimidine) versus ipilimumab. The primary endpoint was immune-related progression-free survival (PFS), which used a modification of the modified World Health Organization criteria, in which the appearance of new lesions does not automatically constitute progressive disease. Unfortunately, the immune-related PFS was only 2.9 months in patients who received ipilimumab versus 4.9 months for patients who continued on fluoropyrimidine maintenance chemotherapy. The median OS was similar in both groups (12.7 vs 12.1 months). Toxicities were also higher in the ipilimumab versus BSC arm (72% vs 56%) and included pruritus (32%), diarrhea (25%), fatigue (23%), and rash (18%).

These 2 studies contain the only data for anti–CTLA-4 antibody monotherapy in EGC (**Table 1**). They suggest modest activity for these drugs at best, and toxicity profiles comparable with the known irAEs of ipilimumab in other cancers.

### Anti–Programmed Death-1 and Programmed Death–Ligand 1 Antibodies

Several anti–PD-1 and anti–PD-L1 antibodies are now approved for the treatment of various cancers. Pembrolizumab, an antibody against PD-1, was initially approved in 2014 for the treatment of advanced melanoma.[22] Since then, it has also obtained approval in non–small cell lung cancer in 2015. In general, toxicities associated with pembrolizumab (and other anti–PD-1 inhibitors) seem to be less than with ipilimumab, as was noted in a phase III study in melanoma that compared 2 doses of pembrolizumab with ipilimumab and found lower rates of grade $\geq$3 toxicities for pembrolizumab (10%–13% vs 20%).[23] The rates of treatment discontinuation were also lower in the pembrolizumab arms than in the ipilimumab arm (4%–6.9% vs 9.4%). Individual grade $\geq$3 toxicities with pembrolizumab were less than 5% and include colitis, hepatitis, and pneumonitis.

Another anti–PD-1 antibody, nivolumab, is also now FDA approved for several malignancies, including melanoma, non–small cell lung cancer, renal cell carcinoma, and Hodgkin lymphoma. Toxicities of nivolumab are qualitatively and quantitatively similar to those of pembrolizumab.[24]

Nivolumab's labeling indication was expanded in 2016 to permit for combination with ipilimumab as first-line therapy for advanced melanoma. This approval was based on a phase III study, which showed improvement in PFS for the combination versus ipilimumab or nivolumab alone.[25] However, this increased efficacy is at the expense of significantly added toxicity (grade $\geq$3 toxicity rate of 55.0% vs 16.3% for the nivolumab arm and 27.3% for the ipilimumab arm).

An interesting observation is that, in patients whose tumors were PD-L1 negative, the addition of ipilimumab to nivolumab improved outcomes compared with

**Table 1**
**Results of anticytotoxic T lymphocyte antigen-4 antibody studies in esophagogastric cancer**

| Treatment | Location/ Histology | No. of Patients | Response Rate, % | PFS Median | PFS Overall | OS Median | OS Overall | Reference |
|---|---|---|---|---|---|---|---|---|
| Tremelimumab | E/GEJ/G adenoCA | 18 | 6 | 2.83 | NS | 4.83 | 33% 1-y | Ralph et al,[20] 2010 |
| Ipilimumab BSC (including chemo) | GEJ/G adenoCA | 57 57 | NS NS | 2.9 mo 4.9 mo | NS NS | 12.7 12.1 | NS NS | Moehler et al,[21] 2016 |

*Abbreviations:* adenoCA, adenocarcinoma; BSC, best supportive care; E, esophageal; G, gastric; NS, not stated.

nivolumab only (PFS 11.2 vs 5.3 months), whereas the addition of ipilimumab did not improve outcomes in patients with PD-L1–positive tumors (PFS, 14.0 months in both groups). This finding gives rise to the intriguing theory that PD-L1 may be upregulated by a tumor as a defense mechanism to dampen the immune system after it has been infiltrated and recognized by T cells. Therefore, in such an inflamed tumor microenvironment, PD-1 blockade alone may be sufficient to exert a significant effect. On the other hand, the absence of PD-L1 inhibition suggests a noninflamed tumor, which requires CTLA-4 blockade to drive T cells into the tumor to facilitate tumor recognition to benefit from blockade of the PD-1/PD-L1 axis.[18]

Finally, an anti–PD-L1 antibody, atezolizumab, was recently approved to treat advanced urothelial carcinoma, based on a single-arm phase II study that treated 310 patients.[26] Toxicities seem to be qualitatively similar to those of the anti–PD-1 antibodies and less than ipilimumab; 5% of patients had a grade $\geq$3 irAE, which included colitis, pneumonitis, and elevation of liver enzymes in 1% of patients each.

Although many of these anti–PD-1 and anti–PD-L1 antibodies have been evaluated in EGC (results are summarized in **Table 2**), only 1 study has been published.[27] The KEYNOTE-012 study is a phase Ib dose-expansion study that evaluated 39 patients with GEJ/gastric adenocarcinomas, whose tumors were found to be PD-L1 positive using an experimental immunohistochemistry (IHC) assay that used the Merck 22C3 antibody. Based on the cutoff for positivity of $\geq$1% membrane staining of tumor or peritumoral mononuclear inflammatory cells, 40% of tumors were noted to be PD-L1 positive.

Nineteen patients were from Asia, and the remainder was from the rest of the world. Patients were heavily pretreated and two-thirds received $\geq$2 prior therapies. The confirmed response rate was 22% for all patients; 4 of these 8 patients had ongoing responses at the time of data analysis, and the median duration of response was 40 weeks. Median PFS was 1.9 months, and median OS was 11.4 months; the 6- and 12-month OS rates were 66% and 42%, respectively. Toxicities seemed to be in line with the known side effects of pembrolizumab and included grade $\geq$3 pneumonitis, pemphigoid, peripheral neuropathy, and hypothyroidism in 1 patient (3%) each.

In the similarly designed KEYNOTE-028 study, 23 patients with PD-L1–positive esophageal cancer were treated, 17 had squamous cell cancer (SCC) and 5 had adenocarcinoma.[28,29] The PD-L1 positivity rate in the screened patients was 41%, virtually identical to the rate in GEJ/gastric adenocarcinoma. This was, again, a heavily pretreated group, with 87% of patients receiving $\geq$2 prior therapies. Seven of 23 patients (30%) had a PR, with 5 of the PRs ongoing at the time of data analysis. The median duration of response was 40.0 weeks. Six- and 12-month PFS rates were 30.4% and 21.7%, respectively.

Nivolumab has also shown promising activity in EGC. Recently, data presented in abstract form suggest similar activity to that of pembrolizumab.[30] Fifty-nine patients with unselected GEJ/gastric adenocarcinoma were treated in a phase I/II study. Eighty-three percent of patients received $\geq$2 prior therapies. The relative risk was 14%, with a median time to response of 1.6 months and duration of response of 7.1 months in the responders. Median OS was 6.8 months for the entire group, and the 12-month survival rate was 36%. PD-L1 positivity was assessed using a cutoff of $\geq$1% for IHC positivity. The relative response rates in patients with PD-L1–positive and PD-L1–negative tumors were 27% and 12%, respectively.

Similar activity was also noted for nivolumab in a Japanese study of 64 patients with esophageal SCC who received a median of 3 prior therapies.[31] PD-L1 positivity was not required nor was it reported in the presented data. The response rate was 17.2%, including a complete response in 1 patient. Median PFS was 1.5 months and median OS was 10.8 months.

**Table 2**
Results of antiprogrammed death or anti–PD-ligand 1 antibody studies in esophagogastric cancer

| Treatment | Location/Histology | No. of Patients | Response Rate, % | PFS Median | PFS Overall | OS Median | OS Overall | Reference |
|---|---|---|---|---|---|---|---|---|
| Pembrolizumab (anti-PD-1) | GEJ/G adenoCA (PD-L1 +ve only) | 39 | 22 | 1.9 mo | NS | 11.4 mo | 6-mo 66% 12-mo 42% | KEYNOTE-012, Muro et al,[27] 2016 |
| | E adenoCA | 23 | 30 | NS | 6-mo 30% 12-mo 22% | NS | NS | KEYNOTE-028, Doi et al,[28] 2015; Doi et al,[29] 2016 |
| | adenoCA | 5 | 40 | | | | | |
| | SCC (PD-L1 +ve only) | 17 | 27 | | | | | |
| Nivolumab (anti-PD-1) | E/GEJ/G adenoCA | 59 | 14 | NS | NS | 5.0 mo | 6-mo 49% 12-mo 36% | Checkmate-032, Le et al,[30] 2016 |
| | PD-L1 +ve | | 27 | | | | | |
| | PD-L1 −ve | | 12 | | | | | |
| | E SCC | 64 | 17.2 | 1.51 mo | NS | 10.8 mo | NS | Kojima et al,[31] 2016 |
| Nivolumab 3 mg/kg q3 wk + Ipilimumab 1 mg/kg q3 wk | GEJ/G adenoCA | 52 | 10 | 1.58 mo | 6-mo 9% 12-mo N/A | 4.8 mo | 6-mo 43% 12-mo N/A | Checkmate-032, Janjigian et al,[35] 2016 |
| | PD-L1 +ve | | 27 | | | | | |
| | PD-L1 −ve | | 0 | | | | | |
| Nivolumab 1 mg/kg + Ipilimumab 3 mg/kg q3 wk | GEJ/G adenoCA | 49 | 26 | 1.45 mo | 6-mo 24% 12-mo 18% | 6.9 mo | 6-mo 54% 12-mo 34% | |
| | PD-L1 +ve | | 44 | | | | | |
| | PD-L1 −ve | | 21 | | | | | |

| Drug | Tumor type | N | Duration | Response | p-value | Reference |
|---|---|---|---|---|---|---|
| Avelumab (anti-PD-L1) | GEJ/G adenoCA (2nd-line) PD-L1 +ve PD-L1 −ve | 20 15 20 0 | 11.6 wk 36 wk 11.6 wk | 3-mo 39% 6-mo 19% 3-mo 60% 3-mo 29% | NS | JAVELIN, Chung et al,[32] 2016 |
| | GEJ/G adenoCA (Maintenance) PD-L1 +ve PD-L1 −ve | 55 7 6.7 3.6 | 14.1 wk 17.6 wk 11.6 wk | 3-mo 54% 6-mo 34% 3-mo 59% 3-mo 44% | NS | |
| Durvalumab (MEDI4736) (anti-PD-L1) | GEJ/G adenoCA | 16 25 | NS | NS | NS | Segal et al,[33] 2014 |
| Atezolizumab (MPDL3280A) (anti-PD-L1) | G adenoCA | 1 100 | NS | NS | NS | Herbst et al,[34] 2013 |

*Abbreviations:* adenoCA, adenocarcinoma; E, esophageal; G, gastric; NS, not stated.

In addition, anti–PD-L1 antibodies also seem to be active. Avelumab produced a response rate of 15% in 20 patients who received it as second-line therapy (although 20% of patients had actually received ≥2 prior therapies).[32] The disease control rate (PR and SD rate) was 50%. Forty-two percent of the 12 tumors in this group that were tested were PD-L1 positive by IHC, using a cutoff of ≥1%. The response rate was 20% versus 0% in the PD-L1–positive versus PD-L1–negative tumors. The median PFS was 36.0 weeks versus 11.6 weeks for PD-L1–positive versus PD-L1–negative tumors.

This study also treated another 55 patients with maintenance avelumab after they achieved a PR/SD on first-line chemotherapy. Four responses were seen (7%), including 1 complete response. Of the 43 patients who had tumor for PD-L1 testing, the response rates were 6.7% versus 3.6% for PD-L1–positive and PD-L1–negative tumors, respectively. Median PFS for the PD-L1–positive versus PD-L1–negative tumors was 17.6 versus 11.6 weeks, respectively.

Finally, abstract presentations also show responses for the PD-L1 antibody MEDI4736 (now called *durvalumab*) in 16 patients with EGC, in which 4 patients had a PR.[33] A PR in 1 gastric cancer patient treated with the anti–PD-L1 antibody, MPDL3280A (now called *atezolizumab*), has also been reported.[34]

The only data for combination immune checkpoint blockade in EGC comes from the Checkmate-032 study, which was recently presented in abstract form.[35] In addition to the 59 patients treated with nivolumab alone (and discussed above), an additional 2 cohorts received different doses of nivolumab together with ipilimumab. Baseline characteristics in these other 2 groups were similar to the nivolumab-only arm. The highest response rate was reported for patients who received nivolumab 3 mg/kg and ipilimumab 1 mg/kg every 3 weeks for 4 cycles (followed by nivolumab 3 mg/kg every 2 weeks), although survival data in these small groups of patients seemed comparable. Grade ≥3 toxicities were also highest in this group (35% vs 5% in the nivolumab arm and 15% in the other arm of ipilimumab 1 mg/kg and nivolumab 3 mg/kg). Nevertheless, this dose has been selected as the basis for a proposed phase III study (see later discussion).

## FUTURE DIRECTIONS

Based on the results above, numerous phase III studies are ongoing or planned, as noted in **Table 3**. Many of these studies are testing similar concepts in the first-, second- and third-line settings for advanced EGC.

Of note, the KEYNOTE-059 study, which has completed accrual, included a first-line arm in which patients received pembrolizumab in combination with 5-fluorouracil/cisplatin. Although efficacy data have not been presented, data presented in abstract form suggested an acceptable toxicity profile for this combination.[36] This combination is being further tested in the phase III first-line KEYNOTE-062 study. The results of both of these studies will therefore determine if there is a benefit for combination immune checkpoint blockade and chemotherapy in EGC.

Also of interest is the Checkmate-577 study, which is evaluating the benefit of adjuvant nivolumab versus placebo in patients with locally advanced esophageal/GEJ tumors (both adenocarcinomas and SCC), who have undergone chemoradiation and surgery but are found to have persistent disease (ypT1-4Nany or ypTanyN+ tumor).

Finally, a phase Ib/II study is evaluating combination immune checkpoint blockade, this time with a PD-L1 inhibitor (durvalumab) and an anti–CTLA-4 antibody (tremelimumab).

These studies represent only a small fraction of ongoing or planned phase I/II studies that will combine immune checkpoint inhibitors with other immunotherapy drugs,

**Table 3**
Ongoing phase II/III studies of immune checkpoint inhibitors in esophagogastric cancer

| Drug | Treatment | Setting | Status | Study Id |
|---|---|---|---|---|
| Pembrolizumab | Pembrolizumab + 5-FU/cisplatin | 1st-line, PD-L1 +ve, Her2 −ve GEJ/G adenoCA | Completed | KEYNOTE-059 (NCT02335411) |
| | Pembrolizumab | ≥3rd-line, PD-L1 +ve or −ve, Her2 +ve allowed if prior trastuzumab GEJ/G adenoCA | | |
| | Pembrolizumab | | | |
| | Pembrolizumab vs paclitaxel | 2nd-line, PD-L1 +ve, Her2 +ve allowed if prior trastuzumab GEJ/G adenoCA | Recruiting | KEYNOTE-061 (NCT02370498) |
| | Pembrolizumab vs 5-FU/cisplatin vs pembrolizumab/5-FU/cisplatin | 1st-line, Her2 −ve, PD-L1 +ve GEJ/G adenoCA | Recruiting | KEYNOTE-062 (NCT02494583) |
| | Pembrolizumab vs irinotecan or taxane | 2nd-line, PD-L1 not assessed, E/GEJ SCC or adenoCA | Recruiting | KEYNOTE-181 (NCT02564263) |
| | Pembrolizumab | 3rd-line, PD-L1 not assessed, E/GEJ SCC or adenoCA | Recruiting | KEYNOTE-182 (NCT02559687) |
| Nivolumab | Ipilimumab 3 mg/kg/nivolumab 1 mg/kg vs nivolumab 1 mg/kg vs chemotherapy | 1st-line, PD-L1 not assessed, Her2 −ve, GEJ/G adenoCA | Planned | Checkmate-649 (NCT02872116) |
| | Nivolumab vs taxane | 2nd-line, PD-L1 not assessed, E/GEJ adenoCA or SCC | Ongoing | NCT02569242 |
| | Nivolumab vs placebo | Adjuvant, PD-L1 not assessed, R0 resection, $ypT_{any}N_{any}$ tumor E/GEJ adenoCA or SCC | Recruiting | Checkmate-577 (NCT02743494) |
| Avelumab | Avelumab vs fluoropyrimidine/oxaliplatin | 1st-line, maintenance, PD-L1 not assessed, GEJ/G adenoCA | Recruiting | JAVELIN-100 (NCT02625610) |
| | Avelumab vs BSC (includes paclitaxel or irinotecan) | 3rd-line, PD-L1 not assessed, GEJ/G adenoCA | Recruiting | JAVELIN-300 (NCT02625623) |
| Durvalumab (MEDI4736) | Durvalumab vs tremelimumab vs durvalumab/tremelimumab Durvalumab/tremelimumab | 2nd-line, PD-L1 not assessed, Her2 −ve, GEJ/G adenoCA | Recruiting | (NCT02340975) |
| | | 3rd-line, PD-L1 not assessed, Her2 −ve, GEJ/G adenoCA | | |

*Abbreviations:* 5-FU, 5-fluorouracil; adenoCA, adenocarcinoma; BSC, best supportive care; E, esophageal; G, gastric; N/A, not available.

chemotherapy, targeted therapies, or locoregional approaches (such as radiation or ablative procedures). Many of these studies are specifically enrolling EGC patients but also include studies that are enrolling EGC patients in dose-expansion cohorts.

## BIOMARKERS OF RESPONSE

The results of the studies discussed above uniformly suggest that less than 25% of patients who receive immune checkpoint inhibitors derive significant benefit. Most studies report a median PFS of less than 2 months, even in the setting of encouraging OS, suggesting that most patients are rapidly progressing on these treatments and that most of the OS benefit may be experienced by the small group who do respond or have disease stabilization. Therefore, the identification of biomarkers to select patients most likely to benefit from these expensive and potentially toxic agents is a priority.

At this time, PD-L1 status by IHC is a leading contender as a biomarker. Although PD-L1–positive tumors seem more likely to respond to treatment with anti–PD-1 and anti–PD-L1 antibodies, many of the studies above suggest the possibility of response and disease control even for patients with PD-L1 negative tumors. Therefore, many ongoing and phase III studies are enrolling patients irrespective of the tumor PD-L1 status.

The situation is further complicated by the fact that there are currently several antibodies available for PD-L1 testing. These antibodies have not been compared against each other to determine if PD-L1 positivity by one test is comparable to the results of another. In fact, there can be issues with reproducibility even using experimental and clinical versions of the same assay[27] and intratumoral and intertumoral heterogeneity and dynamic temporal variability.

Therefore, another possibility is to identify a genetic signature within the tumor and peritumoral tissue that may correlate with an increased chance of benefit from immune checkpoint inhibitors. In the KEYNOTE-012 study with pembrolizumab, a 6-gene signature of interferon-$\gamma$ genes (*CXCL9*, *CXCL10*, *IDO1*, *IFNG*, *HLA-DRA*, and *STAT1*) was assessed using gene expression profiling of RNA isolated from tumor samples to generate a composite score, which was the average of the normalized values of the 6 genes.[27] There was a trend between a higher interferon-$\gamma$ signature score and response, but it did not achieve statistical significance ($P = .070$), possibly a reflection of the small numbers involved (only 30 tumor samples could be tested). One benefit of this gene signature is that it may be more reproducible and robust than PD-L1 testing, and efforts continue to evaluate it in EGC and other cancers.

Finally, there are also ongoing efforts to correlate response and benefit on these studies with the 4 subtypes of gastric cancer, identified by the Cancer Genome Atlas (TCGA) as Epstein-Barr virus (EBV) positive, microsatellite unstable (MSI), genomically stable, and chromosomal instability.[37] Of these subtypes, both the EBV and MSI groups may be more responsive to immune checkpoint inhibition. The EBV subtype accounted for 9% of the tumors in the TCGA analysis and are associated with *CD274* and *PDCD1LG2* amplifications, which encode for the PD-L1 and PD-L2 proteins.

The MSI subgroup accounts for 22% of gastric cancer patients. It is characterized by *MLH1* promoter hypermethylation, which is associated with an elevated mutation rate. A seminal report by Alexandrov and colleagues[38] showed that the prevalence of somatic mutations varies widely among different cancers (**Fig. 2**). The mutation rate is highest in cancers that respond strongly to immune checkpoint inhibition (such as melanoma or bladder cancer), whereas EGC has mutation rates that are less than these cancers but still significantly higher than many other malignancies. Proof-of-principle for this concept comes from activity of pembrolizumab only in

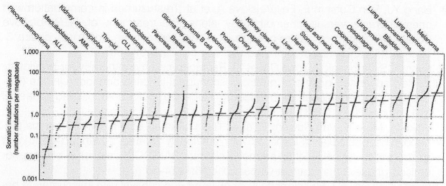

**Fig. 2.** The prevalence of somatic mutations across human cancer types. Every dot represents a sample, whereas the red horizontal lines are the median numbers of mutations in the respective cancer types. The vertical axis (log scaled) shows the number of mutations per megabase, whereas the different cancer types are ordered on the horizontal axis based on their median numbers of somatic mutations. (*From* Alexandrov LB, Nik-Zainal S, Wedge DC, et al. Signatures of mutational processes in human cancer. Nature 2013;500:415; with permission.)

MSI-high colorectal cancer.[39] Recent data also suggest significant activity in other mismatch repair-deficient gastrointestinal cancers, including gastric cancer.[40]

Recapitulation of the TCGA subtypes in a clinical context will be difficult, given that the TCGA analyses were multiplex research tests that required fresh-frozen tissue. However, next-generation sequencing platforms that are now performed semiroutinely in standard clinical care and the IHC characterization of DNA mismatch repair protein status of tumor tissue may permit for the proactive identification of patients more likely to respond to immune checkpoint blockade or to correlate responses with these genetic profiles.

## SUMMARY

The evaluation of immune checkpoint inhibitors in solid tumors in general but also in EGC has occurred at a breathtaking pace. The phase Ib studies that generated significant interest a little more than a year ago have now been overtaken by nearly completed phase III studies.

The results of these phase III studies are, of course, awaited with eager anticipation, and it is hoped that they will establish a new treatment paradigm in EGC, just as these drugs have transformed the treatment of several other cancers. If there is proven benefit for an immune checkpoint inhibitor in EGC, ongoing correlative efforts and the next generation of studies will better delineate the small but significant subpopulation that is most likely to benefit. These efforts will also try to further increase the proportion of patients who will derive benefit by evaluating combinatorial strategies.

In this regard, the many other potential targets noted in **Fig. 1** for antagonist or agonist strategies (many of which are already in phase I/II testing), which can be combined with the current stable of immune checkpoint inhibitors, are a source of promise and a reminder of the significant work that remains to improve outcomes in this difficult disease.

## REFERENCES

1. Ku GY, Ilson DH. Management of gastric cancer. Curr Opin Gastroenterol 2014; 30:596–602.

2. Bang YJ, Van Cutsem E, Feyereislova A, et al. Trastuzumab in combination with chemotherapy versus chemotherapy alone for treatment of HER2-positive advanced gastric or gastro-oesophageal junction cancer (ToGA): a phase 3, open-label, randomised controlled trial. Lancet 2010;376:687–97.

3. Fuchs CS, Tomasek J, Yong CJ, et al. Ramucirumab monotherapy for previously treated advanced gastric or gastro-oesophageal junction adenocarcinoma (RE-GARD): an international, randomised, multicentre, placebo-controlled, phase 3 trial. Lancet 2014;383:31–9.

4. Wilke H, Muro K, Van Cutsem E, et al. Ramucirumab plus paclitaxel versus placebo plus paclitaxel in patients with previously treated advanced gastric or gastro-oesophageal junction adenocarcinoma (RAINBOW): a double-blind, randomised phase 3 trial. Lancet Oncol 2014;15:1224–35.

5. Hodi FS, O'Day SJ, McDermott DF, et al. Improved survival with ipilimumab in patients with metastatic melanoma. N Engl J Med 2010;363:711–23.

6. Robert C, Thomas L, Bondarenko I, et al. Ipilimumab plus dacarbazine for previously untreated metastatic melanoma. N Engl J Med 2011;364:2517–26.

7. Kuby J. Overview of the immune system. In: Kuby J, editor. Immunology. New York: W.H. Freeman; 1992. p. 1–17.

8. Dunn GP, Old LJ, Schreiber RD. The three Es of cancer immunoediting. Annu Rev Immunol 2004;22:329–60.

9. WB C. The treatment of malignant tumors by repeated inoculations of erysipelas: with a report of ten original cases. Am J Med Sci 1893;105:487–510.

10. Karbach J, Neumann A, Brand K, et al. Phase I clinical trial of mixed bacterial vaccine (Coley's toxins) in patients with NY-ESO-1 expressing cancers: immunological effects and clinical activity. Clin Cancer Res 2012;18:5449–59.

11. Old LJ. Cancer vaccines 2003: opening address. Cancer Immun 2003;3(Suppl 2):1.

12. Kantoff PW, Higano CS, Shore ND, et al. Sipuleucel-T immunotherapy for castration-resistant prostate cancer. N Engl J Med 2010;363:411–22.

13. Melero I, Gaudernack G, Gerritsen W, et al. Therapeutic vaccines for cancer: an overview of clinical trials. Nat Rev Clin Oncol 2014;11:509–24.

14. Pardoll DM. The blockade of immune checkpoints in cancer immunotherapy. Nat Rev Cancer 2012;12:252–64.

15. Krummel MF, Allison JP. CD28 and CTLA-4 have opposing effects on the response of T cells to stimulation. J Exp Med 1995;182:459–65.

16. Freeman GJ, Long AJ, Iwai Y, et al. Engagement of the PD-1 immunoinhibitory receptor by a novel B7 family member leads to negative regulation of lymphocyte activation. J Exp Med 2000;192:1027–34.

17. Zou W, Chen L. Inhibitory B7-family molecules in the tumour microenvironment. Nat Rev Immunol 2008;8:467–77.

18. Sharma P, Allison JP. The future of immune checkpoint therapy. Science 2015;348:56–61.

19. Horvat TZ, Adel NG, Dang TO, et al. Immune-related adverse events, need for systemic immunosuppression, and effects on survival and time to treatment failure in patients with melanoma treated with ipilimumab at Memorial Sloan Kettering Cancer Center. J Clin Oncol 2015;33:3193–8.

20. Ralph C, Elkord E, Burt DJ, et al. Modulation of lymphocyte regulation for cancer therapy: a phase II trial of tremelimumab in advanced gastric and esophageal adenocarcinoma. Clin Cancer Res 2010;16:1662–72.

21. Moehler M, Cho J, Kim Y, et al. A randomized, open-label, two-arm phase II trial comparing the efficacy of sequential ipilimumab (ipi) versus best supportive care

(BSC) following first-line (1L) chemotherapy in patients with unresectable, locally advanced/metastatic (A/M) gastric or gastro-esophageal junction (G/GEJ) cancer [abstract]. J Clin Oncol 2016;34:4011.

22. Ribas A, Puzanov I, Dummer R, et al. Pembrolizumab versus investigator-choice chemotherapy for ipilimumab-refractory melanoma (KEYNOTE-002): a randomised, controlled, phase 2 trial. Lancet Oncol 2015;16:908–18.

23. Robert C, Schachter J, Long GV, et al. Pembrolizumab versus Ipilimumab in Advanced Melanoma. N Engl J Med 2015;372:2521–32.

24. Robert C, Long GV, Brady B, et al. Nivolumab in previously untreated melanoma without BRAF mutation. N Engl J Med 2015;372:320–30.

25. Larkin J, Chiarion-Sileni V, Gonzalez R, et al. Combined Nivolumab and Ipilimumab or Monotherapy in Untreated Melanoma. N Engl J Med 2015;373:23–34.

26. Rosenberg JE, Hoffman-Censits J, Powles T, et al. Atezolizumab in patients with locally advanced and metastatic urothelial carcinoma who have progressed following treatment with platinum-based chemotherapy: a single-arm, multicentre, phase 2 trial. Lancet 2016;387:1909–20.

27. Muro K, Chung HC, Shankaran V, et al. Pembrolizumab for patients with PD-L1-positive advanced gastric cancer (KEYNOTE-012): a multicentre, open-label, phase 1b trial. Lancet Oncol 2016;17:717–26.

28. Doi T, Piha-Paul S, Jalal S, et al. Pembrolizumab (MK-3475) for patients (pts) with advanced esophageal carcinoma: Preliminary results from KEYNOTE-028 [abstract]. J Clin Oncol 2015;33:4010.

29. Doi T, Piha-Paul S, Jalal S, et al. Updated results for the advanced esophageal carcinoma cohort of the phase Ib KEYNOTE-028 study of pembrolizumab (MK-3475) [abstract]. J Clin Oncol 2016;34:7.

30. Le D, Bendell J, Calvo E, et al. Safety and activity of nivolumab monotherapy in advanced and metastatic (A/M) gastric or gastroesophageal junction cancer (GC/GEC): results from the CheckMate-032 study [abstract]. J Clin Oncol 2016;34:6.

31. Kojima T, Hara H, Yamaguchi K, et al. Phase II study of nivolumab (ONO-4538/BMS-936558) in patients with esophageal cancer: preliminary report of overall survival [abstract]. J Clin Oncol 2016;34:TPS175.

32. Chung H, Arkenau H-T, Wyrwicz L, et al. Safety, PD-L1 expression, and clinical activity of avelumab (MSB0010718C), an anti-PD-L1 antibody, in patients with advanced gastric or gastroesophageal junction cancer [abstract]. J Clin Oncol 2016;34:167.

33. Segal N, Hamid O, Hwu W, et al. 1058PD - A phase I multi-arm dose-expansion study of the anti-programmed cell death-ligand-1 (PD-L1) antibody MEDI4736: preliminary data, ESMO [abstract]. Ann Oncol 2014;25:iv361–72.

34. Herbst R, Gordon M, Fine G, et al. A study of MPDL3280A, an engineered PD-L1 antibody in patients with locally advanced or metastatic tumors [abstract]. J Clin Oncol 2013;31:3000.

35. Janjigian Y, Bendell J, Calvo E, et al. CheckMate-032: phase I/II, open-label study of safety and activity of nivolumab (nivo) alone or with ipilimumab (ipi) in advanced and metastatic (A/M) gastric cancer (GC) [abstract]. J Clin Oncol 2016;34:4010.

36. Fuchs C, Ohtsu A, Tabernero J, et al. Pembrolizumab (MK-3475) plus 5-fluorouracil (5-FU) and cisplatin for first-line treatment of advanced gastric cancer: preliminary safety data from KEYNOTE-059 [abstract]. J Clin Oncol 2016;34:161.

37. Cancer Genome Atlas Research Network. Comprehensive molecular characterization of gastric adenocarcinoma. Nature 2014;513:202–9.

38. Alexandrov LB, Nik-Zainal S, Wedge DC, et al. Signatures of mutational processes in human cancer. Nature 2013;500(7463):415–21.
39. Le DT, Uram JN, Wang H, et al. PD-1 blockade in tumors with mismatch-repair deficiency. N Engl J Med 2015;372:2509–20.
40. Le D, Uram J, Wang H, et al. PD-1 blockade in mismatch repair deficient non-colorectal gastrointestinal cancers [abstract]. J Clin Oncol 2016;34:195.

# Moving?

## Make sure your subscription moves with you!

To notify us of your new address, find your **Clinics Account Number** (located on your mailing label above your name), and contact customer service at:

Email: **journalscustomerservice-usa@elsevier.com**

**800-654-2452** (subscribers in the U.S. & Canada)
**314-447-8871** (subscribers outside of the U.S. & Canada)

Fax number: 314-447-8029

**Elsevier Health Sciences Division**
**Subscription Customer Service**
**3251 Riverport Lane**
**Maryland Heights, MO 63043**

*To ensure uninterrupted delivery of your subscription, please notify us at least 4 weeks in advance of move.

Printed and bound by CPI Group (UK) Ltd, Croydon, CR0 4YY

03/10/2024

01040401-0014